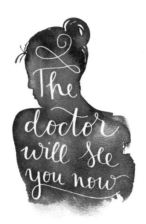

RECOGNIZING AND TREATING
ENDOMETRIOSIS

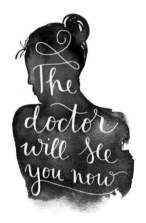

RECOGNIZING AND TREATING
ENDOMETRIOSIS

By Tamer Seckin, MD

TURNER

Turner Publishing Company
Nashville, Tennessee
New York, New York
www.turnerpublishing.com

The Doctor Will See You Now: Recognizing and Treating Endometriosis

Cover design: Nathalie Ouederni and Maddie Cothren
Book design: Kym Whitley
Illustrations: Thom Graves

Library of Congress Cataloging-in-Publication Data
Seckin, Tamer.
 The doctor will see you now : recognizing and treating endometriosis / by Dr. Tamer Seckin, MD.
   pages cm
  ISBN 978-1-68162-112-8 (pbk.)
 1. Endometriosis. 2. Endometriosis--Diagnosis. 3. Endometriosis--Treatment. I. Title.
 RG483.E53S43 2016
 618.1--dc23
                              2015030301

Printed in the United States of America
15 14 13 12 11 10 9 8 7 6 5 4 3 2 1

To the millions of women around the world whose lives are affected by endometriosis, may you find the peace and health you so richly deserve.

Contents

FOREWORD

By Padma Lakshmi

I MET DR. SECKIN in his office in New York in 2006. I had no real hopes that I would hear anything new from what I had always heard from doctors all my life on this visit, so I went with no expectations. But it was this chance, last-minute appointment, which truly changed my life. You see, Dr. Seckin is an endometriosis specialist who has made it his life's calling to treat women with this disease. His thoroughness and care for every single one of his thousands of patients is unmatched. After filling out two detailed questionnaires and going through a thorough physical exam, he told me I had endometriosis and that I would need surgery right away. I had no idea what endometriosis even was, but I realized for the first time, at that moment, that this diagnosis was the beginning of my journey to take back my life.

In 2009, Dr. Seckin and I co-founded the Endometriosis Foundation of America to increase endometriosis awareness, provide advocacy, facilitate expert surgical training, and fund landmark endometriosis research. We knew a lack of disease awareness and misdiagnosis were the two main reasons why so many women suffered for so long. We also knew the medical professionals on the frontline of battling this disease were not properly equipped to diagnose and treat it. It was time for our foundation to lead the charge. To that end, the EFA hosts an annual medical conference welcoming experts from around the world to New York City to meet and discuss the latest research, diagnoses, and treatment options for endo. We host patient awareness days and have created the first school and community-based endometriosis education program. Sales from our latest project, this book, will help fund more outreach programs.

Once diagnosed, I was relieved to know that I wasn't crazy and that there was a reason for all this pain. If you have endo, you're not alone. Having endo has nothing to do with anything you did. It's not because you're weak or a sissy when it comes to pain. You don't have to "buck up" and take it. Endo is not a life-threatening disease, but it does take away your life. Is endo an awful disease? Yes, but changes are happening. There is hope, and there is treatment. Endometriosis doesn't have to be your "lot" in life. There are a lot of things we can't do anything about. But we can do something about endometriosis. If you have this disease or think you might have it, *The Doctor Will See You Now* is a good place to start your road to recovery.

INTRODUCTION

A Letter to you from Dr. Seckin

TO THOSE AFFECTED IN ANY way by endometriosis: I know the pain you've been battling. You hurt, a lot, more than anyone else can comprehend. You feel alone and hopeless. You're physically and mentally drained, nearing your breaking point, if you haven't reached it already. You've tried repeatedly for years to get someone, anyone, to listen to you, to understand what you're going through—a friend, a family member, a school nurse, even a doctor—but they don't. They dismiss your issue as a "girl problem" or a "woman thing," as a disease or condition that it's not, or as something that will magically fix itself over time. They couldn't be more wrong; you know it in your gut, and I know it for a fact. I know it, not due to experiencing this pain myself, but because I was taught by listening to my patients.

To the woman who has had multiple surgeries without symptom relief: You deserve better treatment, and there *is* better treatment. Your doctor is probably giving you the best care he or she has been trained to give, but there are better options that you haven't tried, options that can end your suffering.

To the woman who needs laparoscopic deep-excision surgery but cannot afford it: There are specialists who would be willing to help. You may have to spend more time and resources and conduct more research than you would if you were contending with some other illness, but considering what the results will be compared to the pain you're in now, it will be worth your effort.

To the woman with endometriosis who wants to have a child and is seeking assistance from a fertility clinic, but who hasn't yet become pregnant because the real cause of the problem hasn't been addressed: You can tremendously increase your chances of conceiving a child if the disease is properly treated. Endometriosis is what is blocking your dream, and no fertility treatment can overpower it.

To the adolescent girl who regularly misses school, extracurriculars, and social activities because she is sick but doesn't know why: Yes, you are sick, very sick, no matter what anybody tries to tell you. Just because your girlfriends do not experience the same amount of pain that you do doesn't mean that what you are feeling isn't real. Despite what you have been told, killer cramps are not normal.

To the supportive family member desperately seeking a way to help your loved one who is suffering from endometriosis: I know how difficult this is for you and how much you want to help her. You feel helpless, but please know that she needs your support now more than ever. It's hard for you, but it's worse for her. She's not being dramatic. She really is as sick as she says she is. Together, we can help her get better. But you need to be part of the solution.

To the future doctors whose responsibility it will be to care for patients with endometriosis: We have to work together, not simply to help them get through each day, but to conquer this beast so they can live their lives the way every person deserves to—in peace, comfort, happiness, and without worry or pain. We have to combine the right expertise with an indescribable passion to make them heal. This disease has been debilitating women for centuries. It has to stop now.

And to the woman who has been told by her doctor, family, or friends that she is "crazy," that the pain she feels is all in her head, that it's "not real": It is real. You know it, I know it, the few thousand women I have operated on over the last three decades know it, and the tens of millions of women around the world who have endometriosis know it. You may feel isolated and hopeless right now, but you're not. This book, recounting stories from courageous women who were once in your shoes, will help you see that. It will also give you the knowledge and confidence to advocate for yourself and others from this day forward as together we create a long-overdue awareness about this dreadful disease.

Be well,

Dr. Tamer Seckin

The Disease

1

You're Not Crazy

THE PAIN FROM LAUREN'S FIRST menstrual period ruthlessly attacked her pelvic region. She was thirteen years old. Her friends were going through the same physical changes, which all girls encounter around that age, but their pain didn't appear to be as severe. Lauren could barely get out of bed. When she did, there was no guarantee that she would be able to walk to the next room. She was an excellent student and willed herself to go to school that week, but she became so debilitated that she finally sought help from the school nurse.

Lauren said the nurse believed that eating breakfast would cure her suffering. Lauren knew that was absurd. She explained to the nurse that she hadn't been eating in the mornings because she was nauseous and hurting from the moment she woke up. She knew she would likely vomit any food she ate. The turmoil inside her body wasn't stimulated by a lack of toast or cereal. But her argument was dismissed.

"She just told me to eat more," Lauren said. "And that was it."

I never would have expected anyone in 1990, when this incident occurred, to consider that a girl experiencing such pain during her first period could be on a path toward developing endometriosis. Given that the most respected OB/GYNs in the world knew very little about the disease until the 1980s, there's a good chance the school nurse had never heard of it. But I can assure you that even today, more than a quarter

century after Lauren was told to "eat more," very few people would asso-
ciate her painful period with the possibility that endometriosis could be
developing. Very few would watch for other symptoms of the disease that
might surface. Many women still don't know what endometriosis is. It's
foreign to nearly every man, like just about everything else that occurs in
a woman's body. Believe it or not, even some medical professionals aren't
familiar with this horrible disease or don't know how to properly treat
it. The continued lack of knowledge about endometriosis all these years
later is astonishing but real.

When eating more didn't cure Lauren's ills, and as more symptoms
emerged, including pain deep in the bones and muscles of her legs, Lauren's mother took her to see her pediatrician. And as if the school nurse's
recommendation weren't preposterous enough . . .

"My pediatrician told me I needed to play more," Lauren said. Yes,
play more. Imagine being a vulnerable kid in extraordinary pain, from your
abdominal and pelvic regions down through your legs, and being told *that*
by your doctor. "I couldn't believe it," Lauren continued. "I was a tomboy.
I swam and rode my bike all the time. My mom used to have to come find
me every night because I was so active. And I had to play more?"

How miraculous life would be if eating more and playing more could
mend all our ailments.

As Lauren got older, the pain intensified. In retrospect, it's clear that
endometriosis had manifested itself, but neither Lauren nor anyone else
had any idea that was the cause of her suffering. And, sadly, what little
sympathy she had received steadily decreased. She managed the disease
throughout high school and college either by skipping school on days
when she had her period or by loading up on pain medication before
going to her classes. But when she got her first job out of college and
called in sick each month during her menstrual cycle, that didn't fly with
her boss. "She realized I was calling in sick at the same time every month.
She said, 'Are you not coming in because of your period? You can't miss
work because of your period. We all get it!' She had no idea what kind
of pain I was in."

When bowel issues, kidney and bladder infections, and severe pain
shooting through her spine were progressively added to Lauren's list of
complications, she went to a doctor who administered some tests and ul-

timately did what many doctors who know little or nothing about endometriosis do: he misdiagnosed her with irritable bowel syndrome (IBS). He told her to cut certain foods out of her diet, prescribed her antibiotics, and told her to "drink more water" to help eliminate the kidney and bladder problems. But none of the advice or medication worked because she didn't have IBS. It wasn't much different than putting a cast on the arm of someone with a broken leg.

Lauren went to another doctor to get a second opinion. Actually, a fourth opinion if you count those of the school nurse and pediatrician. Despite the outrageous diagnoses she'd received and false remedies she'd been prescribed over the years, this doctor was at the forefront of insanity—by questioning Lauren's sanity.

"He found nothing wrong with me and said he didn't believe the pain was real," Lauren said. That's right. His professional diagnosis was that the pain that had set up camp in the lower half of Lauren's body and had made her life hell for years was actually sited two or three feet north—in her mind. Telling her to play more would have been better than telling her that. At least the doctor who prescribed Lauren to play more acknowledged that the pain she was feeling existed.

Lauren had never felt so alone. "That's when you start questioning yourself and wondering whether it really is all in your head," she said. "They're either telling me the pain I feel doesn't exist, or they're giving me medicine and advice that aren't working. Nothing made sense to me."

From the age of eighteen until she was about thirty, Lauren took birth control pills to prevent pregnancy. The pain subsided to a small extent while she was on the pill (the pill has been known to provide some comfort to most endometriosis sufferers, which I will discuss in more detail later), but it remained prevalent and continued to have a vice grip on her life. She stopped taking the pill when she and her husband decided to try to start a family, but the pain reached unprecedented levels. From the moment she awoke each morning, the simplest of tasks—getting out of bed, showering, getting into her car—were insufferably difficult. Walking through her office was a genuine test of agility and endurance. When she returned home each evening, she could barely function, let alone be intimate with her husband. Severe headaches kicked in. It was too much to tolerate.

Using the Internet, she researched her symptoms and came to a conclusion that no doctor had ever mentioned as a possibility.

"I went to see my gynecologist and told her, 'I think I have endometriosis,' " Lauren said. "My mom had it, and I was now pretty convinced from what I'd read that I had it." Lauren was six years old when her mom was diagnosed with it. "I remember my mother always being in a lot of pain and very upset, especially around the time of her period," Lauren said. "Because of her, I have known about endometriosis my whole life."

But for a couple of reasons, it hadn't previously occurred to Lauren that endometriosis was causing her trauma. First, neither she nor her mother thought the disease could be hereditary. Second, numerous people throughout her life, including several trusted medical professionals, tried to convince her that it was something else or nothing at all.

And now, the gynecologist rejected Lauren's self-diagnosis, even though it was based on thorough research and extensive experience.

"She said there was no way it was endometriosis," Lauren said. "She said it was such a horrible disease and I didn't have enough of the classic symptoms, so she just gave me more pain medication. But everything I had read about the disease told me I did have it. How much worse could it get?"

Much worse, as Lauren found out one night, not long after seeing that doctor. She and her husband, Tom, hosted a dinner party for a couple of friends and their new baby. Lauren had gotten her period that morning and, as she expected would happen, was not feeling well. But she didn't want to cancel; she was tired of her period dictating her life. Soon after the friends arrived, the baby's mother asked Lauren if she wanted to hold the child.

"She handed me the baby, and I immediately got a sharp stabbing pain in my pelvis," Lauren said. "Holding that baby should have been a beautiful moment, but instead I had to give the baby back to her and excuse myself from the room. I went straight to the bathroom as fast as my body would let me, closed the door, and fell onto the floor in agony. After several minutes, when I still hadn't come out, my husband came in to check on me. He found me in a fetal position, unable to move. 'Can you please ask them to leave?' I cried to him."

Lauren returned to her gynecologist and explained what had happened. The doctor couldn't deny the possibility of endometriosis at this point, right?

Wrong. She did. Lauren was still not symptomatic enough, the doctor said. So she referred her to a fertility specialist.

"It was like my problems were beyond the scope of her experience and she just wanted to get rid of me," Lauren said. "Yes, I was trying to get pregnant and it wasn't happening, but I was more concerned about just functioning day to day. I didn't need a fertility specialist."

Let's pause for a moment and digest Lauren's story so far, which transpired over about twenty years. As a thirteen-year-old, she knew that something was seriously wrong with her body, and she repeatedly sought help from professionals, yet she was continually denied proper care. As the years progressed, she continued to have or developed nearly every classic symptom of endometriosis: painful periods, killer cramps, bowel and kidney issues, pain in her abdomen, pain in her legs, pain in her spine, fatigue, infertility. She also had a hereditary connection: a mother who'd had the disease. Yet Lauren was misdiagnosed numerous times by multiple doctors and, as a consequence, was prescribed useless remedies. One doctor even had the nerve to suggest the pain wasn't real, that it was a figment in Lauren's mind.

Does this infuriate you as much as it does me? Does her plight sound cruelly familiar? Have you experienced any or all of the same frustrations, or do you know someone who has? Two decades had gone by—think about that: an entire generation—and Lauren still didn't have the correct diagnosis or treatment, even after pointedly stating to one gynecologist, "I think I have endometriosis." Unfortunately, the ignorant reactions Lauren received are very common for women with this disease. And because of that ignorance, her torment still wasn't over.

After reading more about endometriosis, Lauren finally decided to see an endometriosis specialist—and the specialist listened! Well, sort of. She concluded that Lauren might have endometriosis, which at least pointed Lauren toward the right path, but the doctor wanted Lauren to go back on birth control pills to see if they would help ease the pain. The pill may have alleviated her pain to a limited extent during the years when she was taking it to prevent pregnancy (she noticed that the pain became more severe when she stopped taking the pill while trying to get pregnant), but it didn't help enough to interest her in going back on it. Lauren wanted surgery and nothing else. She'd already dealt with more pain than most people endure in a lifetime, and she had sufficiently researched the disease to know that surgery was likely her only hope.

The specialist referred Lauren to her partner, who had more experience performing endometriosis surgery. It was eight months before he was able to fit Lauren in, but he finally performed the surgery in January 2012. Lauren was very excited before the procedure because she thought her nightmare might finally be over. But afterward, she reported feeling much worse. "It was terrible," she said. "The pain was unbearable. I had no idea how that was even possible."

It was possible because the doctor had burned off the endometriosis tissue through laparoscopic laser surgery, an ineffective solution. During this procedure—sometimes called ablation, coagulation, or cautery—a heat-producing high-energy source, such as a laser, is used to destroy the part of the lesion that the surgeon can see. (This is different from using a laser to excise the lesion, which I will explain in detail in the chapter on laser surgery.) In general, when I refer to laser surgery throughout this book, I am referring to this "burning off" method, which is done by most surgeons who use laser to treat endometriosis. Laser surgery is not a long-term solution for treating endometriosis, and it's usually not even a short-term one, because doctors are only burning off the surface of the diseased tissue. They are not getting to the root. It's like lopping off the yellow flower of a dandelion without pulling the entire weed, and expecting the yellow flower never to come back. It may look like it's gone, but it's still there, and it will continue to grow and spread until it's properly treated. Laser surgery also leaves behind scar tissue that intensifies the patient's pain. By not removing the disease entirely, laser surgery proves ultimately worse than not performing surgery at all. But Lauren didn't know that. Her doctor didn't either. And Lauren was paying the price.

"Walking was painful just one month after surgery. Sitting down was excruciating. I had an hour's drive to work each day, and I was in tears by the time I got there. I can't believe I never got in a car accident because of how much pain I was in," she said. "I tried to distract myself from the pain as much as I could, but it was impossible. I would come home from work exhausted, and then I'd be up throughout the night because the pain wouldn't allow me to sleep. It was a nightmare."

She'd struggled to walk before the surgery. Now she couldn't even sit without hurting. She didn't know whom else to turn to, so she called the doctor who'd performed the surgery. He prescribed pain medication, but her pain was well beyond that remedy. "It was at about this time that I got a promotion at work, but instead of being happy I wondered how I was going to be able to do the job," Lauren said. "I was in such a bad mental place. I felt like I'd done everything I was supposed to do, but things had only gotten worse."

She didn't give up. She continued to educate herself about the disease and learned about a surgical method called laparoscopic deep-excision surgery. In this procedure, all forms of endometriosis are cut all the way down to the root (as is the thick, surrounding scar tissue) through just a few small incisions made in the woman's body. Laparoscopic deep-excision surgery is performed with the use of very thin instruments, including cold scissors and a laparoscope (a lighted device fitted with a telescopic lens and a miniature video camera). It's a method I have used over the last twenty-plus years and the one I consider the gold standard for removing endometriosis. As I mentioned a few paragraphs earlier, a laser can be used to excise the diseased tissue, but the use of cold scissors yields superior effects. Unfortunately, there are only a handful of doctors in the world with the skill or knowledge to perform this surgery, which is why so few people today—healthcare professionals and patients alike—know about it.

Lauren said, "When I told my doctor who did the laser surgery that there was a procedure that would completely remove the disease, he said, 'If you want to do that, you will have to go elsewhere because I don't do that.'" But even he didn't know where to refer her. It was completely by chance that she found me—while watching a cooking show on television.

"I was watching *Top Chef* one night. I'd never heard of Padma Lakshmi—the host of the show," Lauren said. "Out of curiosity, I got on my computer to find out more about her. That's when I learned she had endometriosis. She talked about Dr. Seckin and what he'd done for her. His method of cleaning out all the endometriosis was exactly what I was looking for. It just seemed to make perfect sense."

Lauren lived in New Jersey, about an hour from my Manhattan office. She called me, and we met about two weeks later. When she came in, we discussed everything she had endured since her teenage years. She hadn't personally known a single person who had experienced what she'd been through; her mother's pain with endometriosis wasn't nearly as severe as her own experience with pain. I, on the other hand, knew a few thousand women just like her—women I had successfully treated. After a long, candid consultation during which we earned each others trust, I conducted a thorough physical exam on her, including a rectovaginal exam, and I could feel the endometriosis inside her. There was no doubt in my mind that every symptom she had—back pain, leg pain, side pain, kidney infections, migraines, difficulty sitting and standing, you name it—was caused by the endometriosis.

"It just seemed like he understood me and believed me right from the outset," Lauren said. "I couldn't believe that with one meeting and one exam, he was able to tell me what was going on and that he knew how sick I was. I couldn't even get some doctors to believe that I was in any pain at all."

I also invited her husband, Tom, into my office so I could explain her condition to him. No man will ever know the physical pain associated with endometriosis, but when his spouse or partner is going through it, he certainly experiences the emotional strain with her. Although a woman who has a partner may occasionally come into my office by herself, she usually brings her significant other for support, which I always encourage. Her partner has been emotionally suffering with her for as long as they have been together, and they come to me as a team, both of them more than ready to end the agony. The disease limits their sexual activity. It can prevent them from having children. It can affect their financial situation because she may be unable to work. It can ruin their social life. All these obstacles can create rifts within a marriage or partnership that can be difficult to overcome.

"I felt helpless as a partner," Tom said. "I wanted to help her, but I never could. I would hold her hand, but all I could say to her was that the best I could do was take her to the ER. That was hard."

"It was very difficult for my husband to go through this. I was a very cranky and crabby person for a long time," Lauren said. "And meeting with Dr. Seckin was very hard on him. It was tough for him to hear just how sick I was and that there was nothing he could do himself to make me better. But he never gave up on me. All he cared about was me being happy and well."

We scheduled Lauren's surgery for November 2, 2012. Nothing short of a natural disaster was going to stand in her way of getting this done. In fact, even that wasn't going to stop her. Less than a week before the surgery, Hurricane Sandy rocked the East Coast. "We didn't have power for a week," Lauren said. "I couldn't use the phone. I couldn't reach the doctor's office. I was freaking out! Finally, they were able to reach me the day before the surgery and told me that if I could get to Manhattan, they'd do it. I told them I'd crawl there if I had to!"

Lauren made it (without having to crawl!), and the surgery lasted nearly six hours. She had endometriosis everywhere. And I mean everywhere. With quite a bit of difficulty, I had to tilt her uterus, remove the cyst, reconstruct her ovaries, put the uterus back in place, and maneuver my way through the thick scar tissue that had formed as a result of the previous doctor's laser surgery. It was one of the worst cases of endometriosis I'd seen in a long time. But I was confident when I was finished that I had excised it all.

"I woke up to Tom holding my hand," Lauren said. "I felt instantly better. The next day I was able to sit up in my bed and look out the window without any pain at all. It had been years since I had been able to do that. It felt like the first day of a new life."

But Lauren would have to deal with one more bit of heartache, one last sucker punch from the endometriosis before starting that new life.

"It was always my dream to go into federal law enforcement, specifically with the US Postal Inspection Service, one of the top placements for federal law enforcement," she said. "It was very difficult to get in, but I'd made it through the initial testing period, polygraph, and background check. All I had left to get through was a four-month training camp. They called me to go through the camp just two weeks after my surgery. I was still recovering and couldn't do it that soon."

Unfortunately, they only give you one opportunity.

"I still think about it because it was tough to let go of something I really wanted," she said. "I've worked as a property manager for the last eleven years, and I love my job, I really do. But knowing my dream is never going to happen is difficult. It's not like I didn't study enough; my body just let me down."

Lauren and her husband had also wanted children at one time, and I think it could have happened after the surgery with the aid of fertility treatments, but the thought of putting her body through that was not one she wanted to entertain. And who could blame her after the twenty-five years of hell she'd endured?

Yet today, Lauren is one of the happiest people you could ever meet. She is active in endometriosis support groups; she is flourishing in a career she loves; she says she is "95 percent" pain free; and her relationship with Tom, whom she has been with since age fifteen, just two years after she was first struck with the symptoms of this disease, is strong as ever.

"Life is great," she said with conviction. "My day-to-day quality of life is unreal. The pain is not even a thought anymore. I can drive to work. I can walk. I don't have to cancel family events. Tom and I just try to laugh every day and have a good time with each other. What more could I ask for? I felt so hopeless, and now I want to make sure other women have hope and know there are doctors out there who can help."

I'm fortunate to have so many patients who, like Lauren, are willing to courageously share their personal journeys. Their stories can help reassure you that although you or someone you know might have this disease, there is hope. I included Lauren's story first because it represents the many textbook cases I've encountered. It encompasses practically everything a woman with endometriosis could go through: physical pain at a very early age; multiple symptoms; multiple misdiagnoses; a lack of understanding, knowledge, and experience on the part of doctors who she thought could help her; a doctor who told her the pain wasn't real; years-long inner turmoil caused by not knowing what was wrong with her; a laser surgery that didn't work and even made her feel worse; a career path shut off to her—and the ultimate solution, deep-excision surgery with cold scissors, that finally ended her misery.

Lauren's bravery and her determination to defeat endometriosis are typical of all the women I treat. Other things they have in common are an initial lack of knowledge about the disease and how it should be treated —and the fact that they've consulted doctors, often more than one, who also lack knowledge about the disease and how to properly treat it. The lack of awareness about a condition that has debilitated millions of women throughout history must end.

The women suffering from this insidious disease want better. They deserve better. It's time to help them—to help you—conquer it.

2

The Road Less Traveled

Two roads diverged in a wood, and I—
I took the one less traveled by,
and that has made all the difference

THE LAST FEW LINES OF Robert Frost's poem "The Road Not Taken" have always resonated with me. There are two roads: one leads to established studies and treatments for well-researched diseases; the other is a treacherous, unexplored road. It leads to ailments of the human body that require treatments still unknown to us. Endometriosis stands among them. In the field of gynecology today, there is still no allocated academic training for treating this disease exclusively. Early in my gynecological career, I recognized that significantly more attention needed to be dedicated to endometriosis. This observation is what drove me to do what I do today. I am told that I am an expert in this field at a level few doctors can match. I accept this praise with absolutely no narcissism. It's a statistical fact—one that I want to change, and one that must change. This shouldn't be a class of just a few. Imagine if only a handful of doctors knew how to treat heart disease, cancer, or diabetes. We need more doctors to have the knowledge, determination, and devotion to help the millions of women who have endometriosis—from those suffering today to the baby girls being born right now who will begin experiencing symptoms in a little more than a decade.

Before I delve into explaining what endometriosis is and everything associated with it (symptoms, misdiagnoses, treatments, etc.), I want to tell you about myself so I can earn your confidence like I do with all my patients, and like every doctor in every aspect of medicine should do with all of his or her patients. Once that trust is established, I believe it will help you comfortably discuss endometriosis with others as you seek treatment or as you support someone you know while she seeks treatment.

I was raised in Turkey and attended a very progressive all-boys boarding school founded by American missionaries in Tarsus (the birthplace of St. Paul). My first assignment from my father when I left home for Tarsus at age eleven was to read the autobiography of Albert Schwietzer. Schweitzer was a musician and a missionary doctor, and he became my greatest inspiration, particularly considering his commitment to healing his patients. In December 1967, two years after I began boarding school, the first human heart transplant took place in Cape Town, South Africa. I read several news reports on how Dr. Christiaan Barnard accomplished this tremendous feat. I was obsessed with the superhuman agility, precision, and speed that Barnard's hands must have possessed to accomplish something that seemed impossible at the time. I knew that his naturally skilled hands performed the surgery not due to magic, but rather because of dedicated hard work and hours of repetitive technical improvement.

I started medical school in 1972 in Ankara, Turkey, and I knew immediately that I wanted to pursue the surgical field. I have always been a very visual person, and a very curious one. My first experience using laparoscopy to visualize the inside of a woman's pelvis occurred when I was an intern at medical school. That same year, I was one of the first doctors in Turkey to use a fetoscope, a thinner version of a laparoscope. Attempting to see a fetus inside the amniotic sac deeply moved me.

I came to the United States in 1980 and trained for five years in Buffalo, New York, before moving to New York City to work for other doctors. I've often been asked why I chose New York, one of the most challenging cities in the world in which to work, given its huge population and the fierce competition it engenders in just about every field. But that's exactly why I did it: for the challenge. I had the privilege of observing the works of Dr. Camran Nezhat and working side-by-side with Dr. Harry Reich, a pioneer in the detection and treatment of endometriosis. Both of these doctors have been my mentors and good friends. Dr. Reich discovered, along with others, that the disease could be better diagnosed and treated using the minimally invasive laparoscopy surgery as opposed to the much more invasive laparotomy surgery, in which a large incision is made in the abdominal cavity. He recently retired as one of the top laparoscopic surgeons in the world. I started my own practice in 1987. Starting my own practice was not my original plan, but after years of encountering so many women suffering from pelvic pain and often finding no relief, it was something I strongly felt I needed to do.

In my years of training and working for other doctors before Dr. Reich, part of me believed that the practice of gynecology was misleading patients concerning the subject of pelvic pain. The misleading was not intentional; it was due to inherited and preconceived practice patterns in the field of gynecology. Women were dragging themselves into gynecologists' offices in disastrous physical and mental states. They often had no idea what was wrong with their bodies and sought any sliver of hope they could find. But they left with none. Nobody could help them. In fact, the women themselves were often blamed for their problems, and because they were being blamed by an "expert," these women left believing their doctor, or at least they didn't openly question their doctor.

During my residency training in Buffalo, pelvic inflammatory disease was the reason given for practically all pelvic pain experienced by women. Pelvic inflammatory disease is caused by an infection of the reproductive organs by bacteria that are often transmitted sexually. We checked for gonorrhea, chlamydia, or herpes. If the tests came back negative, we'd simply say, "We're sorry, but we couldn't find anything wrong." We, as licensed doctors, were judging them based on their sexual health. We insinuated that their pain was contracted from sexual intercourse. Because of our own blindness concerning the cause of their pain, we assumed that they were hiding their sexual history from us, that they were not telling us the truth. That bothered me—a lot.

Back then, endometriosis was not well known. The understanding of every disease must begin somewhere, and we had barely cast a light on this one. In fact, it was not until the late 1980s that a more specific definition and diagnoses of the early stages of the disease began to surface. Dr. David Redwine and Dr. Dan Martin, who were practicing from Oregon and Tennessee, respectively, defined early endometriotic lesions as being differently colored than normal, healthy tissue. Today, it is known that endometriosis lesions are varied in color, appearing as black, brown, red, blue, white, and even clear. At the time, however, the truth behind this disease concerning women's pelvic pain was only beginning to become more apparent.

I believed then that there was more to endometriosis than what we saw. So much more that we should know and practice. There was no way all those women in pain were lying about their conditions. That's what triggered my focus on this disease. These women needed serious help, and they weren't receiving the proper care. I couldn't fall in line with practices that started centuries ago, as you will read about in the next chapter. There had to be a new approach. There had to be an answer, and I was convinced we were missing it.

I saw gynecology—and, specifically, endometriosis—as a very challenging field. I saw it as something deep, vast, unbelievable. I know those are not adjectives people usually use when describing gynecology, but the exploration into the unknown, with the potential to end a woman's years of suffering, captivated me. My work fighting this disease—from doing surgeries to advocating the power of early diagnosis to promoting research for prevention and a cure—has been laborious, but it's been worth every second because I see light at the end of what has been a very long and dark tunnel.

In 2006, with the support of a growing number of patients whom I had successfully treated, I was encouraged to create a grassroots foundation to bring more recognition to endometriosis. I filed for 501(c)(3) charity status for the Endometriosis Foundation of America (EFA), and Padma Lakshmi graciously accepted my offer to be the cofounder. The EFA, which officially launched in 2009, is the first research and advocacy foundation of its kind organized by a private physician to raise awareness about the disease and emphasize the critical value of deep-excision surgery. In 2010, I organized the first EFA Medical Symposium, now an annual event. The conference brings together the top surgeons and scientists from around the world to speak to and train the next generation of medical professionals. That year, with Dr. Elizabeth Poyner, I also started the Fellowship in Minimally Invasive Gynecologic Surgery in affiliation with the American Association of Gynecologic Laparoscopists/Society of Reproductive Surgeons at North Shore/LIJ-Lenox Hill Hospital in New York City, where I am also the Clinical Instructor for Obstetrics & Gynecology.

In 2012, I received the Ellis Island Medal of Honor for my work as a philanthropist and women's health advocate, and for establishing the EFA. I was also named one of America's Super Doctors by *New York Times Magazine.*

I have worked as an executive officer for the International Society of Gynecological Endoscopy, which has afforded me the privilege of traveling around the world to give lectures about my experience treating endometriosis, and to perform surgeries at Lenox Hill Hospital that are transmitted live by satellite to China and various countries in Europe.

I am currently working with the Feinstein Institute for Medical Research on a genetic research initiative to create the first endometriosis tissue bank in the United States, and I'm also a member of about a dozen other national and international organizations focused on women's reproductive health.

Again, I'm sharing all of this with you so you feel comfortable with who I am and with my expertise in tackling the disease that has a stronghold on you or on a loved one. I want you to understand the experiences of Lauren, Annie Rose, Nicole, Laura, Jessica, Sara, Padma, and the rest of the two dozen women whose incredible journeys with endometriosis you will read about, and I want you to know that you are not alone.

I have performed about three thousand laparoscopic surgeries in my career, removing an average of eight to nine endometriosis lesions in each case, amounting to the removal of more than twenty thousand lesions. These have nearly all been minimally invasive laparoscopic surgeries, almost scar-less procedures. I have taken the road less traveled for women in pain who are searching for answers, knowing that current and future doctors will join me in the effort to eliminate this horrendous disease. I have taken that road with the belief that women diagnosed with endometriosis can candidly discuss their symptoms and help us create a public awareness that will bring relief to other suffering women. And it is my conviction that, in the end, together we will have made all the difference.

3

Endo What?

WHEN A DOCTOR INFORMS A patient that she has diabetes, high blood pressure, heart disease, cancer, or some other common malady known to the general population, the patient will more than likely have an idea of what the condition is and what she will have to do to treat it. Treatment may require a change in diet, exercise, medication, chemotherapy, surgery, or some combination of these. A patient's subsequent knowledge of the disease stems not only from the number of people affected by the illness, but also from the awareness about it that has been raised through years of educating the medical community and the public.

If the public's knowledge of a disease were purely based on the number of people who were diagnosed with it, everyone would know about endometriosis. At least 10 percent of American women of childbearing age have endometriosis.[i] Yet when I tell one of my patients that she has it, the first words out of her mouth are often the same words I heard from Padma when I diagnosed her: "Endo what?" The public still lacks awareness of the condition. Lauren was a rare exception because her mother had endometriosis. If Lauren's mother hadn't had it, Lauren might still, to this day, be wrestling with an undiagnosed disease. She wouldn't even have visited the first specialist she saw because she wouldn't have known to. No previous doctor had mentioned the term *endometriosis* to her. Her mother was the one who made her aware of it.

Consider these statistics:

- An estimated 176 million women worldwide suffer with endometriosis, according to an article in the *Journal of Endometriosis and Pelvic Pain Disorders.*[ii]
- The disease takes, on average, nearly twelve years to diagnose in the United States and roughly eight years to diagnose in the United Kingdom, according to a survey published in the journal *Human Reproduction.*[iii]
- The American Society for Reproductive Medicine says endometriosis can be found in up to 50 percent of infertile women.[iv]
- An article in *Human Reproduction* states that direct healthcare costs of endometriosis and indirect costs of time lost from work due to endometriosis amount to an estimated $110 billion annually in the United States.[v]
- According to a recent Finnish study that appeared in the *Journal of Pediatric & Adolescent Gynecology*, one-third of girls ages fifteen to nineteen were found to suffer severe menstrual pain, of which 14 percent were consequently regularly absent from school or hobbies.[vi]

Numerous women have endometriosis but don't know they have it. And those who do know they have it often don't talk about it. Why the silence? Several reasons. There's the taboo that still exists against anything involving a woman's menstrual period; the exhaustion of being repeatedly misdiagnosed; the stigma of always being sick—the list goes on, and it will be discussed in greater detail in subsequent chapters.

So what is endometriosis? My description will be simple and comprehensive, so much so that any person, even those who are ignorant about how the female body works, will understand it.

Endometriosis is defined as the presence of endometrial-like tissue outside of the uterine cavity. By "endometrial-like tissue," I mean tissue that greatly resembles the endometrium, which is the interior lining of the uterus that grows every month to prepare the uterus for the implantation of a fertilized egg. Endometriosis causes pelvic pain in reproductive -age women and adolescent girls and is associated with heavy menstrual periods, clotted flow, gastrointestinal symptoms, fertility problems, and a tremendous loss of quality of life.

Throughout the ancient and modern history of endometriosis, doctors and researchers have had different theories and opinions as to what causes it. Just recently we learned that endometriosis can be present at birth; it was found in some newborn fetal autopsies and was attributed to the fetuses' exposure to elevated levels of maternal pregnancy hormones, namely estrogens and progesterones. The belief is that although a female may have endometriosis at birth, it doesn't activate until her first menstrual period. I believe the disease can be inherited, as you will read about in the chapter on genetics. Many also believe, that the disease can be caused by retrograde menstruation. While this is a controversial view, my thirty years of clinical observation suggests that retrograde menstruation must play a triggering role in the development of endometriosis, particularly through the gene material in the stem cells. It is likely that the disease may actually occur differently in different women, allowing for multiple hypotheses, which is why I offer the opinion of Dr. Harry Reich in Chapter 39. Research investigations have yet to provide clear answers.

"Retrograde" means "moving backward." Retrograde menstruation refers to a woman's menstrual blood flowing back into her body during her period. Let me explain further. Ovulation—the hatching of eggs from the ovaries—occurs in a woman's body each month. Fourteen days later, if there is no pregnancy, she has her menstrual period, during which her body naturally sheds the endometrium. If the menstrual flow properly exits from her body, the flow carries the endometrium with it through the cervix, the opening of the uterus that connects to the vagina. The cervix is small, strong, and tight; it opens to allow menstrual blood out, but it also keeps a baby in the uterus for nine months. When the labor starts, uterine contractions dilate the cervix to allow the baby into the vaginal canal for the birthing process.

If the menstrual flow does not exit as it should, the menstrual blood may leak back into the body through the natural openings in the fallopian tubes. Where does menstrual blood go? It implants in areas outside of the uterus in the pelvis and creates an abnormal growth of cells: endometriosis cells with inflammation. That's not a good thing, and it may get worse. The body's immune system desperately and futilely tries to eliminate these dislocated cells, which results in deeper inflammation with new blood vessels and stem cell activity resulting in deep and thick scar tissue. As a woman's hormones (estrogen and progesterone) change during her menstrual cycle, the implants (which are also called lesions or nodules) respond to the hormonal fluctuations by growing. In other words, estrogen and progesterone are feeding the beast, serving as food for the implants. Unfortunately, unlike the endometrium that naturally leaves the body, there is no way for the implants to exit the body, so the inflammation continues.

This is endometriosis—menstrual periods that are literally stuck inside of a woman's body. The implants can grow deep and wide, spreading and clinging to her uterus, appendix, rectum, ovaries, intestines, leg nerves, and other parts of the pelvic region. They are like leeches that attach to, reproduce on, and grow on whatever internal organs they find. They are similar to a slow-growing cancer that invades the organs in the pelvis. In some rare cases, they can spread to the diaphragm, lungs, kidneys, or brain.

The disease always causes inflammation, which can lead to adhesions, scarring, internal bleeding, bowel or urinary dysfunction, constipation, painful intercourse, and infertility. The physical pain can be unbearable, which inevitably leads to psychological pain. A woman's career may suffer. Relationships with loved ones may become strained. She may have to miss a lot of school, or even drop out. This disease threatens to become a woman's identity, ruling every phase of her life.

Endometriosis, however, is a treatable disease. Some of my patients say that the deep-excision surgery I performed on them "cured" them. Although they may feel as though they are cured—because I was able to remove all their endometriosis and, as a result, transform their lives to the extent that they are pain-free and happier than they have been in many years—there is no guarantee that the disease won't return at some point. The hope is that it won't, but it could. Endometriosis is not like a bacterium you can eradicate with antibiotics or a virus you can prevent with immunization. It's something that can continue to happen to some women's bodies throughout their lives, and it needs to be recognized, diagnosed, and eradicated by excisional removal each time.

Whether one believes that the disease is curable or incurable, it is at the very least treatable through deep-excision surgery, and many women who undergo the surgery can reclaim their lives and live pain-free, which is a significant advancement from days of old.

The history of endometriosis dates back centuries and is believed to be tied to misdiagnoses of hysteria, which is defined in part by Merriam-

Webster as "a state in which your emotions are so strong that you be-
have in an uncontrolled way." It's telling that the word hysteria comes
from the Greek word for uterus. The use of hysteria to mean uncontrolled emotions arose from the ancient, outdated notion that *hysteria*
was unique to women and resulted from disturbances of the womb. In
a brilliant article about the origins of endometriosis that appeared in the
Journal of Fertility and Sterility in 2012, Drs. Camran Nezhat, Farr Nezhat, and Ceana Nezhat write:

> By applying this broader set of criteria we were able to uncover substan-
> tial, if not irrefutable, evidence that hysteria, the now discredited mystery
> disorder presumed for centuries to be psychological in origin, was most
> likely endometriosis in the majority of cases. If so, then this would consti-
> tute one of the most colossal mass misdiagnoses in human history, one that
> over the centuries has subjected women to murder, madhouses, and lives of
> unremitting physical, social, and psychological pain. The number of lives
> that may have been affected by such centuries-long misdiagnoses is stagger-
> ing to consider, likely involving figures in the multiple millions.[vii]

Take a moment to digest that. "One of the most colossal mass misdiagnoses in human history" with "multiple millions" of lives affected.
Women subjected to murder and madhouses. Have you heard of any
other disease described that way?

Another article, written by the *Associated Press* and published in the
New York Times on December 5, 2012, states that famed neurologist Sig-
mund Freud diagnosed female patients with hysteria when he could not
determine another diagnosis:

> It is surmised today that hysteria at the time Freud diagnosed it was more
> closely related to the manner in which a woman reacted to her pain and
> symptoms rather than to the actual cause of her pain. Through extensive
> research and in-depth analysis doctors today believe that what Freud may
> have diagnosed as hysteria was really endometriosis.
>
> Diagnosis of hysteria, witchcraft and demonic possession were com-
> monplace during the time Freud was diagnosing patients. Treatment mo-
> dalities included administration of noxious substances, hanging women

upside-down, and enduring painful surgical procedures that included a physician using his fingernail in place of a scalpel long before anesthesia had been discovered.[viii]

Demonic possession and witchcraft? You can blame "the times" as an excuse; they didn't know then what we know today. Recall from Chapter 2 one of the reasons why I began focusing on this disease early in my career: because I knew that the women we couldn't diagnose weren't lying to us, and I knew they deserved better treatment. Technology has improved immensely. Research is better. But has the attitude toward endometriosis and toward the pain these women endure really changed much? Back to the article in the *Journal of Fertility and Sterility:*

> [W]hat we can say with reasonable assurance is that endometriosis appears to be an old disease that has affected women for millennia. Allusions to its insidious presence are documented in ancient medical texts dating back more than 4,000 years. That endometriosis appears to have such an ancient lineage makes it all the more surprising that it is, for the most part, still an enigma. Perhaps most remarkably, some treatments have remained the same for hundreds of years with only minor variations.[ix]

And it is "still an enigma." Here in the twenty-first century, women such as Lauren are still being told their pain isn't real, or that it's being caused by something else. Such an archaic reaction in today's medically advanced world doesn't seem possible, but it's happening globally and every day to women with endometriosis. At least no doctor ever suggested to Lauren that she was possessed by the devil or that she should be hanged upside down, though given some of the astonishing stories my patients have told me about their experiences with previous doctors, nothing would surprise me.

Think about the number I cited early in the chapter: an estimated 176 million women worldwide are believed to be affected by endometriosis. That's roughly the equivalent of every single female in the United States having it, regardless of age. Along with being a leading cause of infertility and chronic pelvic pain, endometriosis has also been linked to other health concerns, including certain autoimmune diseases, fibroids, adenomyosis, interstitial cystitis, and even certain cancers. Businesses lose billions of dollars each year in reduced productivity because of this disease. It is also one of the leading reasons why doctors perform laparoscopic surgeries and hysterectomies in the United States, which I will address soon.

Recent studies list other theories about factors that may cause endometriosis, including genetics, immune disorders, metaplasia (a cell's ability to change into another type of cell more suited to its new environment), and exposure to environmental toxins. Any woman can develop endometriosis, but there is a strong belief evolving in the medical community that some patients may be genetically predisposed, such as Lauren may have been. It is believed that a woman who has a mother or sister with endometriosis is about six times more likely to develop the disease herself, and that lesions may actually start implanting in her body soon after she is born. Studies also suggest that the risk of developing it is higher for women who get their period at an early age, experience heavy periods, have periods that last more than seven days, or have monthly cycles of twenty-seven days or fewer.

One of the most frustrating aspects of this disease is how long it can take for a woman to be properly diagnosed. On average, a woman is twenty-seven years old and has had endometriosis for a decade before she is diagnosed with it, a result of the lack of education about the disease among healthcare professionals and the general public. Diagnosis of endometriosis in its early stages—preferably immediately when the pain starts, but even within months or a year instead of a decade—will literally change the course of a woman's life.

Diagnosing endometriosis requires three steps. First, a clinical exam and testing (such as a sonogram and/or an MRI). Second, visually identifying the lesions through laparoscopy. Third, a pathologic exam of the lesions under a microscope. I have been doing this long enough to know after the clinical exam whether or not a woman likely has endometriosis. In fact, sometimes I can tell from the moment she comes into my office by the way she walks or how she shifts her body when she sits. But until I can see inside her through laparoscopy, I don't know how extensive it is—what organs or other parts of the abdominal and pelvic cavities it is affecting.

All forms of endometriosis can be associated with significant pain and infertility; early intervention is the key to resolving the disease and its devastating effects. If Lauren had been diagnosed as a teenager rather than in her late thirties, not only would she have avoided all that physical pain, but she possibly would have earned her dream job in federal law enforcement and had children. Endometriosis dictated the path of Lauren's life, placing significant limits on her potential for fulfillment and happiness.

Another patient of mine, Sara, remembers her pain beginning when she was about fifteen, and it took nearly fifteen years more for her to be diagnosed. "It got progressively worse the older I got," Sara said. "In my midtwenties it was really bad. By my late twenties, it was unbearable. I was getting urinary tract infections every other month. I had a hard time digesting food. My face and body would swell. If I didn't have pain meds, I would be on the floor in a corner unable to do anything. It was just so painful all over. I told my OB/GYN how painful my periods were, and his solution was for me to take more Advil. There was never a thought from my doctor that it could be something bigger."

But there absolutely should have been. That mentality must change in the people these women count on, especially doctors and other health-care professionals.

In upcoming chapters I will impart additional valuable information about endometriosis: the stages of the disease; the symptoms; the misdiagnoses; the effects of having it; the treatments that will help a woman manage it so she can live a normal, healthy life. I will also describe ongoing efforts to educate people about the disease, and what the future holds for today's prepubescent girls who will one day experience it.

But first, I want to talk further about the pain caused by this dreadful illness, and I want to introduce you to more incredibly strong women who've tolerated that pain day in and day out. If you are a woman who does not have this disease, or if you are a man, understanding the level of pain that can result from endometriosis will help you empathize with someone who does.

NOTE: See images 2A, 2B, and 3 in the photo section starting on page 93.

4

Pain, and its Effect on Personality

ENDOMETRIOSIS–SPECIFICALLY, THE PAIN IT produces—shapes many patients' attitudes, states of mind, and personalities. Because the pain is real, it affects the brain, and can change its functions. For this reason, I think of some of my patients as having "Type E personalities," with the E standing for endometriosis. Type E personalities are women who will not allow any outward signs of their pain to show as long as they can help it. Some endometriosis patients have the ability to block their pain despite the distress it causes them. They will wake up at six o'clock in the morning, grab their coffee, get the kids out the door, go to work or school all day, attend meetings or social functions, close business deals, take exams, care for their families and homes, play with their kids, then do it all again the next day. They will painfully, but silently, suffer through their daily activities, refusing to show any weakness. They're tough. They don't want anyone to know what they are battling inside.

In 2015, at the annual medical conference I host for healthcare professionals, Dr. Sawsan As-Sanie, with the University of Michigan Health System, stated that the brain's perception of continuous pain causes visible changes in neural networks and brain morphology as seen in MRIs. This results in the rewiring of our midbrain, which is responsible for creating changes in our inner persona. That chronic pain and consequent rewiring is what causes a woman's personality to change.

"Having endometriosis is horrific, but it proves how physically and mentally strong you really are," said Jessica, one of my patients. "Yes, it takes an extreme toll on your body and mind, but when you can say, 'Okay, I handled this,' you know that you can handle absolutely anything." Endometriosis can affect the personalities of the women who suffer from it—all due to pain, and the specific, unique, and entirely different ways in which patients cope with pain.

So what is pain? Pain is real. It's something that is felt. It is the brain's perception that something wrong is happening with the body. It's an instinctive vital sign. As a physician, pain is a very believable aspect of a patient's condition. If a person says she is feeling pain, then there is pain. I have to believe her. I cannot be judgmental about that in any way. Considering all the hell that Lauren went through, what bothered me more than anything else about her story was that a doctor once told her it was all in her mind. I've had many women tell me that they've been told the same thing by their doctors. Why would a woman who says she is feeling pain, especially in such a personal and private area of her body, make up something like that? All doctors need to respect pain.

A woman with endometriosis, when she reflects on her journey with the disease, usually realizes that the pain began with her very first period. A girl that age who is developing endometriosis will experience excruciating pain, unlike anything she has ever felt in her young life. I would say I have found that to be the case in at least 90 percent of my patients. But because it's her first period, she doesn't necessarily know it should not be that painful. If she says something about it to her mother, her father, her sister, her teacher, her friends, or even her doctor, she is usually told, "This is normal. This is just how it is moving into womanhood." She is told she has to smile and bear it. What she is not being told is what's not normal. Normal is a relative term, but when a girl is in that much pain from the start of her menstrual cycle, someone in authority should recognize that something out of the ordinary is wrong. Unfortunately, and unbelievably, that rarely happens.

So the young girl accepts the pain because she's been told to, and she lives with it every day, even as it gets progressively worse. She will likely not mention it to anyone again, at least not for many years, until she is older and more independent. One reason is the taboo factor that exists with respect to women's periods and their symptoms. Every woman has menstrual periods, but every woman experiences a different level of pain. She doesn't hear other women complain, so she's not going to either. She does not want to be labeled as weak or as a whiner. She doesn't want to be teased about it. She accepts what she was originally told by her mother or doctor about its normalcy, takes a couple of ibuprofen, and deals with it. That shapes her mental attitude toward the pain as the intensity increases with each period.

"I remember in school going to typing class and being doubled over from the pain during my menstrual period," said Annie Rose, a patient from New Jersey. "But I never missed a day of school. I fought it. I was constantly worried because I would bleed through my uniform. My parents would bring me a new skirt because I bled into the other one. I was called horrible names by kids for that. But I never missed a day." Annie Rose was willing to tolerate bleeding into her clothes and getting bullied, as long as she didn't miss a day of school.

Elissa, a single mother of three from New Jersey, had a multitude of endometriosis symptoms for years: irregular periods, killer cramps, constant stomach pain, diarrhea, lightheadedness, blurred vision, and severe back pain. She also had a miscarriage and underwent several surgeries by another doctor, including a hysterectomy that I believe was probably not necessary, before she came to me. She had to hold on to the furniture when walking through her house or taking care of her young children. She spent four hours on the road every day—a two-hour commute to and from work—which equaled the amount of sleep she got each night. Her parents and a few friends helped her when they could, but Elissa had always been a very independent person, never the type to ask for help. Having endometriosis didn't change that about her.

"Honestly, I don't know how I did it. I just did it," she said. "I had kids. I had work. I had responsibilities that I needed to take care of. You feel like a zombie just going through the motions, but you have to do what you have to do. I especially did it for my kids because I didn't want to scare them or have them worry that something was wrong with me." She said she learned to get used to the pain, and she even became immune to some of it. "It's kind of like when you smell a skunk," Elissa said. "Your initial reaction is 'Oh, wow!' because the smell is so sudden and strong. But then you breathe it in, let your olfactory senses get used to it, and you move on."

Eventually, though, the pain can push every woman to her breaking point. It may take years, but it can happen.

The physical pain caused by endometriosis comes in several varieties. There's painful periods, chronic pelvic pain, pain during intercourse, painful bowel movements, rectal pain, and urinary pain. Besides pain, there can be nausea, vomiting, diarrhea, constipation, and migraine headaches. Sometimes a woman can experience several symptoms at the same time, an all-out attack.

Before Padma Lakshmi was referred to me by a physician named Dr. Ronald Primus, she had been to some of the most renowned gynecologists in the world, from New York to California and across Europe, but left each doctor's office in the same state she entered: in constant, unbearable pain, and with no hope in sight. In one instance she underwent an appendectomy after a doctor thought that might be the fix. It wasn't. Another doctor extracted a cyst from one of her ovaries, but the pain persisted with a vengeance.

Padma's physical suffering began after her first or second period when she was thirteen years old. The monthly routine that followed was debilitating: severe cramps and excessive bleeding for about seven days, being bedridden for at least three of those days, and being in "very considerable pain" the other four. Her physical ailment gradually developed into a mental misery that plagued every fiber of her soul. She was thirty-six years old when I first met her; she had been suffering for more than two decades.

"When I say 'very considerable pain,' what I mean is that my boobs hurt and my butt hurt. My back hurt and my legs hurt. And my stomach hurt. And my head hurt. Most of all my heart hurt," Padma said during a talk she gave at one of my medical conferences. "My mother, who was a nurse and a very educated woman, told me that she suffered from many of the same symptoms, and that some girls got it and some girls didn't. This was my lot in life."

Padma tolerated her condition and managed the best she could throughout high school and college, but doing so came with a steep price. She missed several days of school each month and many significant family events, she had to change her clothes multiple times a day during her period because of the bleeding, and she habitually took heavy pain medication just to be able to function.

"And, along the way, I went to regular checkups," she said. "It is always a pain in the ass and elsewhere to go to a gynecologist, but it was especially so for me because I would tell them what I had and they would just say, 'Yes, yes.' They would kind of nod their heads in sympathy and prescribe more pain medication. I could not understand why I did not get to just take a couple of Advil and pop in a Tampax and go on about my day. When something has to do with such a deep part of your womanhood, but your body and your sexuality are abnormal, that pain—emotional and physical—just radiates outward. It makes you wonder if the rest of you is normal at all, or will be."

Her pain and bewilderment continued after college and lasted well into her professional career. "I started working as a model in Europe—in Paris and Milan—and there were a lot of times when I had to cancel jobs," she said. "There were a lot of times when I had to cancel personal trips, vacations, and a lot of times when I just did not want to tell people why, because it is really embarrassing to talk about your period, especially when you are a young girl. It is really not fun. Not to your boyfriend, not to the editor who has hired you for the lingerie job, not to anybody, really." And so she did what Type E women do: she accepted it and continued pushing forward.

Laura, a thirty-five-year-old patient from New Jersey, knows the pain all too well. She began menstruating when she was thirteen. The cramps that came with her period were nothing out of the ordinary. Her body was changing. She knew that. But around her sophomore year of high school, the cramping became unduly painful, so agonizing that her cycle included two to three missed days of school every month. The living room couch was her sanctuary during those dark times. Heating pads and over-the-counter pain medications were her teddy bears. She did not think this was normal, until a doctor told her it was. "I went to an OB/GYN who said that sometimes women have these things and that I just had to deal with it," Laura said. "That made sense to me and I accepted it."

Liza, a patient from Brooklyn, clearly noted her painful periods on the initial paperwork she filled out when she went to see her gynecologist.

"They gave me a form, I checked that I had painful periods, and they never asked me a single question about them when I got into the exam room," Liza said. "I wondered why they didn't ask me any follow-up questions, but I never asked. I just assumed that everyone must have painful periods, and that was the end of it."

The physical agony these women tolerate is just the beginning of their torment. Consistent pain, particularly when repressed, can eventually cause lasting emotional distress. And the way in which doctors, friends, and family treat the woman who is suffering can cause her further mental anguish. In part, this process explains the history of the disease's misdiagnosis over the decades and centuries. To repeat a sentence from the 2012 *Associated Press* article quoted in Chapter 3: "It is surmised today that hysteria at the time Freud diagnosed it was more closely related to the manner in which a woman reacted to her pain and symptoms rather than to the actual cause of her pain." In many cases today, that line of thinking has not changed.

"I went to seven gynecologists, and they all said the same thing: they couldn't find anything wrong with me," said Annie Rose, the woman who was doubled over in typing class as a teen and refused to miss a day of school. You've heard of patients being diagnosed with something and wanting a second opinion. Imagine going for a third opinion, a fourth, a fifth, a sixth, a seventh . . . and receiving virtually the same opinion each time, all of them wrong! For women with endometriosis, this happens quite often. Annie Rose was twenty-five years old when she saw that seventh doctor. It was her fourteenth year of torture. "One gynecologist told me he was sick of hearing me complain, and he told me to go home and think about what was causing my pain. He thought it was depression."

Nicole, a psychologist and patient of mine, had excruciating abdominal pain on the first day of her cycle most months beginning in her teen years. The pain intensified with time. It was bad in high school and college, worse in her early twenties, and debilitating in her thirties. She'd been diagnosed with endometriosis in her midtwenties, and doctors tried to treat it in the years following with several laser surgeries and birth control pills. But any pain relief that resulted from those treatments was temporary.

"I was at work one day and was in so much pain that I ended up in a fetal position on the floor," Nicole said. "I struggled to get up and walk long enough to get to my car in the parking lot." When she finally reached her car, she drove herself straight to the emergency room.

"I was kept overnight for observation and tests, but all the tests came back negative," Nicole said. "None of the doctors wanted to address the real issue, which was endometriosis. I felt frustrated, misunderstood, and helpless."

Before she was discharged, she asked the gastroenterologist on duty if there was pain medication she could take. He said he would refer her to a pain medication specialist, but he also threw in his two cents, a comment that just about sent Nicole through the roof.

"He said that sometimes antidepressants are helpful," she said. Yes, he said that to a licensed psychologist. "I can't tell you how livid I was. I just can't imagine all the women out there who are begging for someone to help them end the physical suffering this disease has inflicted upon them, but who are told that the pain is psychosomatic."

These women are not crazy. They know it, I know it, and everybody needs to know it. They need someone to listen to them. Someone to believe their pain is real. Someone who will say to them, "This is not normal." Someone who can fix them and return them to a normal physical and mental state. In fact, they don't just need one person, but multiple surgeons, physicians, friends, and loved ones who want to help remove this disease.

In 2012, after seven doctors had let her down, I successfully operated on Annie Rose. It was one of the very few times going into a surgery in which I wasn't sure how successful I would be given how widespread her endometriosis was. But today, Annie Rose's pain is nearly completely gone, and she has regained full mobility in her left leg.

"I'm a fighter, and I encourage other women to hang in there and trust their bodies," Annie Rose said. "If a doctor says you have endometriosis, do not wait to get it treated. Go see a specialist immediately. And if someone tells you there is nothing wrong with you but you know there is, or if someone tells you there is something mentally wrong with you but you know it's physical, trust yourself."

Symptoms

5

From Early Endo to a Frozen Pelvis

THE SCIENCE BEHIND ENDOMETRIOSIS IS quite fascinating to me, but I know that most people battling the disease or who know someone battling it care primarily about getting answers to three questions, and in layman's terms: What is endometriosis? What is it doing to my body? What do we need to do to get rid of it? The old adage "Give it to me straight, Doc!" applies to most people. Patients want to have a clear understanding of the disease and what they can or should do to treat it, but they don't necessarily need or want to know every nuance or scientific term that relates to it. To help provide them with that understanding so that they can seek proper treatment, here is some pertinent information on the stages of the disease.

Endometriosis is classified into four stages by the American Society for Reproductive Medicine: I (minimal), II (mild), III (moderate), and IV (severe). Criteria for determining those stages are based on the location of the endometriosis, the extent to which it has spread, the depth of the endometriosis, the presence and size of ovarian endometriomas (more on those in just a moment), and the presence and severity of adhesions. A point system determines the stage a woman is in. It has been revised three times in the past forty or so years to reflect the continued progress we have made in learning about the disease. A score of one to fifteen indicates minimal or mild endometriosis (stage I or II). A score of sixteen or higher indicates moderate to severe endometriosis (stage III or IV). However, the point system and the four stages have no specific correlation to any symptoms and exclude the infiltrative nature of the disease. That means the level of pain a woman is in plays no role in determining which stage she is in. So someone with stage IV (severe) endometriosis may feel little or nothing at all, while someone with a stage I (mild) case could be seriously hurting.

When I talk to my patients about the location and severity of their endometriosis, I discuss the four stages, but sometimes I refer to a slightly different, more descriptive system that also features four classifications: early endometriosis, ovarian endometriomas, deep infiltrating endometriosis (DIE), and frozen pelvis.

Early endometriosis is also called minimal peritoneal endometriosis, or peritoneal disease. Almost all endometriosis starts in the peritoneum of the pelvis. The peritoneum is the membrane that lines the abdominal cavity. Peritoneal disease often shows no symptoms at all, including any pain. If there are symptoms at this stage, they are usually most severe in adolescents and will include gastrointestinal distress such as nausea, vomiting, and diarrhea.

The peritoneum is a pristine organ—a shiny, transparent, slippery, delicate, thin layer that separates the pelvic organs, bladder, kidneys, and parts of the colon from the rest of the abdomen. In early endometriosis, the peritoneum of the pelvic area will not show any gross anatomical distortion during a laparoscopic exam because the disease is in such an early stage. This is why visual recognition and identification of early endometriosis is a must for proper treatment. A doctor cannot treat endometriosis, or any disease, if he or she cannot recognize it and identify it. Because endometriosis is so difficult to see, a very close inspection is necessary. This involves bringing the camera to near contact with the peritoneal surface. During the exam, many textural changes will be visible in differently colored implants (pigmented lesions). Red lesions are the youngest lesions. They usually look like miniature grapes with capillary blood vessels sprouting from them. These sprouting capillaries are the earliest form of endometriosis lesions; their growth is known as angiogenesis. As these capillaries rupture, their colors change to violet and black. White lesions are usually the coverings of these underlying active and deep lesions.

Increased surface tension can be easily recognized. The implants could cause chronic recurring bleeding and inflammation, which could lead to fibrosis (thickening and scarring of the areas affected by endometriosis). So, ultimately, what starts as early endometriosis could become moderate to severe peritoneal disease that includes the disfiguration of organs and the pelvic anatomy.

When I see angiogenetic activity sprouting from the surface of the peritoneum, and when I recognize the development of new vessels at the capillary level, I am astonished at how they resemble the clear and bright stars in the night sky. Like the stars in the universe, we have vague ideas on how these endometriosis lesions came into being. And we are astonished by how small we can be made to feel on account of their immense power.

Treatment for peritoneal endometriosis is the primer excision surgery aimed at removing both the lesions and the collateral damage caused by inflammation. During this excision surgery, I use the "ABC" technique that I developed. *ABC,* or *aqua-blue contrast,* refers to the blue-tinged water I introduce into the affected area, which enhances the visibility of lesions that are difficult to see (occult lesions) due to the overpowering brightness of the laparoscopic light source. Using the ABC technique, I can recognize about 30 percent more lesions and wide areas of inflammatory texture changes in the peritoneum. Otherwise invisible lesions become visible. It's like stars in the sky during the day are not seen due to very bright sunlight. When the sun's light disappears at night, the stars and heavens come into view. In a similar way, the ABC technique eliminates the bright laparoscopic light, allowing the surgeon to discern endometriosis lesions otherwise not visible.

Ovarian endometriomas are highly common and may be present in 30 to 40 percent of women with the disease. Endometriomas are large, fluid-filled cysts that form on, and may even encapsulate, the ovaries. They are comprised of menstrual debris, including fragments of endometrial tissue, thickened blood, and inflammatory enzymes. Also called "chocolate cysts," because of the color of the old blood they contain, they can rupture, causing their contents to spill and cling to the walls and the nearby organs in the abdominal cavity. That glue-like fluid can cause excruciating abdominal and pelvic pain. In patients with an ovarian endometrioma, the symptoms and sonographic findings are often dismissed by general practitioners who assume the woman has nothing more than a simple cyst. They will often tell the patient there is nothing to worry about. But if that chocolate cyst ruptures, I believe there will be plenty for the woman to worry about.

I treat ovarian endometriomas through laparoscopic cystectomy. This involves removing the lining of the cyst and reconstructing the ovary. As I do this, I temporarily suspend the ovary in the peritoneum so that it does not stick to the pelvic sidewalls. The removal of the ovarian cyst must be done with precision and without compromising the ovary's blood supply. After an ovarian cystectomy for endometriosis, patients are prone to having diminished ovarian function due to the loss of ovarian follicles. I try to reduce that possibility by following meticulous techniques using microsurgical principles. I do not use any electricity during ovarian surgery (to avoid "frying" the eggs). I use sutures rather than electric coagulation. When I do surgery, it is rare that removal of the ovaries (called an oophorectomy) is necessary to remove endometriomas. An oophorectomy should be considered only if there is a suspicion of cancer, continued persistence of the disease, or severe adhesions that could cause neuropathy (nerve damage).

There are two types of deep endometriosis. One is called **deep infiltrating endometriosis,** or **DIE,** an invasive form of the disease that is often characterized by the penetration of the bladder and the bowel wall. The other, which is the more common form of deep endometriosis, is **deep fibrotic nodular endometriosis.** These nodules distort the entire anatomy in the cul-de-sac, the area between the uterus and rectum, without invading the bowel and bladder walls. The cul-de-sac encompasses the rectovaginal septum (the space between the vagina and rectum), the uterosacral ligaments, the pelvic sidewall, and the bladder. When deep endometriosis infiltrates pelvic sidewall nerves, it causes neuropathy. Both types of this significant and severe form of endometriosis are strongly associated with high levels of pelvic pain, painful bowel movements, painful sex, anatomic distortion, infertility, leg pain, and intestinal distress such as gassiness, bloating, constipation, or diarrhea. My surgical treatment for DIE is the same as that for frozen pelvis.

Frozen pelvis is horrific. All the stages are awful in their own ways, but this one is the worst. Pelvic organs are partially or totally cemented. Frozen pelvis is the most extensive form of advanced endometriosis, encompassing the most extreme forms of deeply infiltrative endometriosis. This aggressive form of the disease includes everything described in the three previous classifications, along with unusually deep infiltrative attachments to the outer limits of pelvic ligaments, nerves, and muscle tissues. Deep fibrotic nodules and deeply infiltrative endometriosis replace pelvic soft tissues with high-density fibrosis. Pelvic organs become firmly glued to pelvic bones, making the pelvis fully or partially frozen and immobile. It's similar to the way it would feel if a block of concrete were stuck inside the pelvis. Although most stages of endometriosis are diagnosed based on viewing the pelvis during surgery with laparoscopy, an experienced endometriosis surgeon can easily diagnose frozen pelvis during a pelvic exam in the office.

Here is a more detailed, easy-to-follow explanation of how frozen pelvis can occur: Endometrial tissue can implant on and invade any part of the body, and it does so most frequently in the peritoneal cavity of the pelvis. Remember, the peritoneum is the lining that separates the pelvic organs, bladder, kidneys, and parts of the colon from the rest of the abdomen. Endometrial implants are tissues similar to the tissue that lines the inside of the uterus. Therefore, they are affected by and subjected to a similar reaction to the hormones estrogen and progesterone. That reaction is to bleed. In other words, mini menstruations occur at the sites of these implants as the hormone levels fluctuate during a woman's monthly cycle. Unlike a period, however, the menstrual bloodshed from these lesions becomes trapped in the peritoneal lining, while the immune system fights to clear the debris that results from the trapped bloodshed. The outcome of the struggle between the two forces is inflammation. The inflammation ultimately results in increased scarring, or adhesions. These adhesions can "glue" internal organs together, wrap around organs, form web-like structures from organ to organ, or attach to the peritoneum. All this activity produces a lot of pain. When a surgeon looks at the peritoneal cavity and sees adhesions stretching from the ovaries to the fallopian tubes, to the pelvic sidewalls, and to the cul-de-sac, he or she knows this may be just the beginning of a much more serious problem. The adhesions may extend to deeper tissues involving the nerves, lymph nodes, and/or muscle layers of organs. After the adhesions dig deeper, they harden soft tissues and organs in the pelvis. What started as an early peritoneal implant becomes a rock-like tissue due to fibrosis.

If the thought of implants on your organs having mini menstruations, of your organs being glued together, or of your organs being entangled in web-like structures doesn't make you squirm, then I don't know what will. People often have the attitude that if something bad is out of sight, then it's out of mind. Why even think about it if we can't see it? But women suffering from severe endometriosis cannot get it out of their minds because they feel it every second. It cripples them. This is the devastating power of the disease.

My first step during a pelvic exam of someone with frozen pelvis is to feel for a firmly fixed uterus. Sometimes the frozen tissues involve nerves and blood vessels in both the front and back of the uterus. As I perform a vaginal exam, a patient who has frozen pelvis will feel extreme pain since the pelvic organs have lost all their flexibility and the adhesions are pulling on other organs. Usual functions such as a bowel movement, emptying the bladder, menstruation, and sexual intercourse are extremely painful due to the restrictive nature of scarring and the altered anatomy. Bowel obstruction, kidney swelling, ureter swelling, and bladder dysfunction are frequently caused by frozen pelvis.

In addition, there are several outward symptoms of frozen pelvis. The patient may experience severe leg pain or pain in the sciatic nerve around the time of her period. She may be unable to cross her legs, or even sit due to pain in her tailbone. Most patients with frozen pelvis complain of severe changes in bowel habits, possibly including constipation, diarrhea, painful bowel movements, and a gassy and bloated feeling. Patients also experience frequent urination, difficulty holding urine (caused by decreased bladder capacity), and flank pain (pain around the kidneys) caused by an obstructed and dilated ureter. Most patients at this stage of endometriosis have also stopped having sexual intercourse because the disease is located in the upper part of their vagina. Sex would be incredibly painful for most endometriosis patients. It is also common for pain to continue for several days after sex. Often, all these symptoms occur together.

When diagnosing frozen pelvis, I follow the initial office exam with an endovaginal sonogram. The primary purposes of the sonogram are to rule out any other diseases within the uterus and to rule out any presence of an endometrioma in the ovaries. A rectovaginal exam is the last part of the office evaluation. I check for nodules in the rectum and upper vagina. After that, I send the patient for an MRI of the pelvis so that I can see the depth of the endometriosis and the status of the kidneys, ureters, and bladder.

Surgery for frozen pelvis is, as you might imagine, an intense team effort. It can last more than six hours. Along with me in the operating room will be a urologist, a colorectal surgeon, and a vascular surgeon if needed. All of us are specialists in our fields as advanced laparoscopic surgeons.

There you have it: the stages of endometriosis. The important thing to note is that no matter what stage you are in, your condition needs to be treated, and sooner rather than later. The disease must be detected and treated with precision at pixel resolution, which is offered by a high-resolution camera. The endometriosis surgeon must utilize the most meticulous techniques, avoid energy sources when possible (which can cause thermal damage to tissue or damage the eggs when operating around the ovaries), and be able to do the fine suturing that is necessary. If the surgeon is uncomfortable going through the walls of organs, such as the bowel and bladder, diseased tissue will be left behind, and the symptoms will persist and become worse.

The longer the condition is left untreated, the more it will spread, and the greater potential there will be for more vital organs and the patient's overall quality of life to be affected. This is why it's important to know the symptoms, to respect them when you recognize them, and to get the proper diagnosis and treatment as swiftly as possible.

NOTE: See images 1A, 1B, 4, 5, 6, 7, 8, 9, 10A, 10B, and 11 in the photo section starting on page 93.

6

The Taboo of Periods

THE MOST DIAGNOSTIC CLUE OF endometriosis, what I call "the first cardinal symptom" of the disease, is painful periods. In Chapter 3, I explained the theory of retrograde menstruation. The menstrual period is almost always when the pain begins for a victim of this disease, and it often begins with her very first one as a young adolescent. I would never diagnose a thirteen-year-old girl with endometriosis based solely on painful periods, no matter how much they hurt, but such a complaint would certainly prompt me to look for other possible symptoms that could confirm that the disease was materializing. Painful periods are a cardinal symptom in adolescents that are accompanied by intestinal distress such as gassiness, nausea, and vomiting. These symptoms have a peritoneal origin and are most likely caused by irritation due to retrograde bleeding.

A major hurdle in diagnosing endometriosis early in a woman, as I've briefly mentioned, is the taboo of talking openly about periods. The vast majority of my patients had exceedingly painful periods beginning with their very first one, but they didn't say anything to anybody when the pain initially started because they were too embarrassed, they didn't realize the pain was abnormal, or they were shunned by doctors or their loved ones when they did say something. As a result, they didn't speak about the subject, choosing instead to live with their condition. A painful period is the first cardinal symptom of endometriosis, yet it's often ignored simply because of what it is.

I strongly believe it is the responsibility of adults to educate adolescents, girls and boys, about menstrual periods. In fact, I'd say it's a necessity if the stigma is to have any chance of being broken and if we are going to have any chance of consistently catching this disease at its onset in women rather than after they've suffered for years. Girls and boys should be taught what periods are, the physiology behind them, and how they are as natural to women as the changes that male adolescents go through. The conversation with a boy will likely be neither very long nor very emotional. It doesn't have to be. But the stigma surrounding a woman's period cannot be broken if males are not part of the conversation. Males' attitudes toward periods, which can include unflattering jokes or simply trying to avoid the subject altogether, are a major cause of the stigma, and education can help erase that—especially if young males learn that the condition could be affecting their grandmothers, mothers, sisters, or, eventually, daughters.

Adolescent girls should additionally be taught what to expect when they get their first period, when they should expect it, and the best ways to handle it, physically, emotionally, and socially. They should be invited to ask questions, and they should expect to be able to get the answers they seek and need without fear of embarrassment. They should be encouraged to track their symptoms and to discuss them with a gynecologist who will listen. The adults who educate girls on this topic can be anyone, including fathers or male doctors. Given what I do for a living and my knowledge of the subject, I can talk about periods with my daughters the way many fathers can talk about sports with their sons. Sometimes it's even dinner conversation in my house! But a significant female in a girl's life, someone she trusts wholeheartedly and who has gone through or is going through the experience, is the ideal person—a mother, a sister, an aunt, a grandmother, a guardian, or a close friend. As is the case in most situations, the best education and awareness will come from those who have the most knowledge, experience, and understanding.

The person imparting the advice should not put the burden of responsibility on the girl by waiting for her to come forward and ask questions, because that may not happen. For example, if we're talking about a girl's mother, she should observe her daughter's behavior and attitudes to know if physiological changes are likely occurring in her daughter. The mother should pay close attention to her daughter's schoolwork, sports activities, engagement in hobbies, and relationships with friends and family. How is her daughter behaving? What is her attitude? Are problems arising in school or with others that weren't there previously? Everything needs to be approached with tenderness, confidence, and complete understanding, as starting her period is likely the biggest physical and hormonal change to date in the daughter's young life.

Of course, this is all easier said than done. In some cultures, periods are still seen as very dirty. There are countries today in which any woman of any age who is going through menstruation is banished from her community until her period has passed, or she cannot touch certain things, such as food, that others might touch. It's difficult to believe this sort of thing happens in the twenty-first century, but anything is possible with a lack of scientific education.

In March 2015, an author and artist named Rupi Kaur did a project titled *period* for a course in visual rhetoric at the University of Waterloo in Ontario, Canada. She and her sister, Prabh Kaur, took a series of photos that showed a woman having her period. The photos included a side view of a woman lying down in bed with blood on her clothes and sheet, blood in a toilet, an overhead view of blood on a shower floor between the woman's feet, and a woman lying down holding a hot water bottle on her pelvic region. Rupi wrote this beautiful prose:

i bleed each month to help make humankind a possibility. my womb is home to the divine. a source of life for our species. whether i choose to create or not. but very few times it is seen that way. in older civilizations this blood was considered holy. in some it still is. but a majority of people. societies. and communities shun this natural process. some are more comfortable with the pornification of women. the sexualization of women. the violence and degradation of women than this. they cannot be bothered to express their disgust about all that. but will be angered and bothered by this. we menstruate and they see it as dirty. attention seeking. sick. a burden. as if this process is less natural than breathing. as if it is not a bridge between this universe and the last. as if this process is not love. labour. life. selfless and strikingly beautiful.[xi]

Little did Rupi know the worldwide outrage that her project would spark, which perfectly proved the point of the project. Rupi posted one of the photos from the series on the social media site Instagram. The photo caused such a stir that Instagram removed it. Rupi responded by reposting the same image an hour later. After Instagram removed the photo a second time, Rupi shared a screenshot of the notification she'd received from Instagram about the photo being removed. Beneath the screenshot, Rupi expressed her concerns about Instagram's actions. She also expressed her frustration through a post on Facebook, which went viral. As the story of the removed photo spread rapidly throughout the world, Rupi received angry messages, including death threats, from people who saw her photo and were appalled by it. Eventually, Instagram apologized to her, and both photos were restored.

In an article that appeared in the *Huffington Post* about Rupi's project and the global reaction to it, Rupi explained her inspiration. She said that she wondered why she always tried to hide her tampons and pads from people, and why she was too ashamed to tell people about the pain her periods caused her. "Why do I lie about it?" she said. "As if it's a *bad* thing to have."[xii]

Rupi also told the *Huffington Post* that she had endometriosis. Starting a discussion about the disease itself was not the primary point of her project, but she indirectly brought tremendous awareness to the condition by focusing on the root of why so few people know or talk about it: because of the taboo of menstruation. Rupi is an artist and poet first, but she is also a pioneer in trying to end the stigma around discussing a woman's period. This discussion needs to continue, and we *all* need to realize that we have a role to play in that.

A woman who is suffering from painful periods needs to speak up, but she needs to be educated at an early age to know that she should speak up. When should she say something? How much pain is normal? How much is too much? How long does a normal period last? How much blood is normal? Again, *normal* is a relative term. If a woman bleeds profusely for several days, if she suffers from debilitating pain in her pelvic or abdominal area during her period month after month—so debilitating that she can't walk, go to school, or do her job—and if the pain lasts more than a couple of days or persists after her period, it is definitely something she should consult a doctor about. If the pain is strong and there are other symptoms with it, such as gastrointestinal symptoms, vomiting, diarrhea, painful bowel movements, back pain, or leg pain, it is also probably something that should be examined. She needs to feel confident that if she does speak up, someone is going to listen to her and understand what could be wrong. That is the responsibility of parents, husbands, teachers, counselors, nurses, and doctors.

The one simple and straightforward question that every female should be asked when she consistently suffers from agonizing pain, but one she is rarely asked, is "Do you have these symptoms with your period?" All doctors should ask that question, including pediatricians, who have known most of their patients since they were babies. If you have a friend or mother or daughter or sister who you think may have endometriosis based on what you have read so far, ask her that one simple question about her pain: "Do you have these symptoms with your period?" If the answer is "I don't know," have her track her symptoms over a couple of months. If the answer is "yes," give her this book. After years of her suffering and feeling hopeless, you may have just helped put her on the road to a proper diagnosis and effective treatment.

7

Killer Cramps

LIGHT CRAMPS DURING A PERIOD are normal. They may feel uncomfortable, but an over-the-counter pain medication should take care of the problem well enough to enable a woman to go about her day. But killer cramps, the second cardinal symptom of endometriosis, are not the "normal" kind of cramps. These cramps are frequently associated with very heavy and prolonged menstruation, and the blood is usually clotted. Killer cramps are of uterine origin in adolescents, but in later years, because the disease spreads to different areas, they are signs of more advanced endometriosis. The pain from killer cramps is so severe, so intense, that it completely alters a woman's daily life. She may have to stay home from work, school, or other activities, and for days at a time. She may not be able to play with her kids or drive them to their appointments. She may have to excuse herself in the middle of a social function and find somewhere private to lie down so that she can catch her breath and try to mentally get through the episode. She may not even be able to get out of bed to begin with. Killer cramps kill whatever she is doing or wanting to do at the time. They aren't just a nuisance that she has to deal with, like normal cramps. They take over her life. They become in charge of her.

This symptom correlates with the first cardinal symptom of painful periods. The reason I list them as two separate symptoms is because painful periods can include more than killer cramps. When Lauren had her period and collapsed on the bathroom floor after holding her friend's baby, she was experiencing killer cramps, but it went well beyond that. Her endometriosis was so invasive that the sharp pain she felt resonated throughout her entire pelvic area and into her legs.

Killer cramps may start out feeling like normal cramps, but the level of pain suddenly and quickly escalates to an incapacitating level. They can happen not only during menstruation but also during ovulation.

Eve became a patient of mine in the mid-1980s when I worked with another doctor, and she remained with me when I started my own practice in 1987. She was around thirty years old when she initially came to see me, and she had been suffering with undiagnosed endometriosis for years. She displayed a few different symptoms of the disease. Though she experienced very little bleeding during her periods, she suffered extreme leg pain. The worst symptom she faced was cramps. She started getting them with her first period at age thirteen. They would last a full three days. "I can close my eyes right now and remember them like they happened yesterday. I will never forget them," Eve said. "The pain would literally knock me off my feet. I did go to school because my mother made me go; she didn't believe me that it was that bad. She never had a pain in her life. Sometimes she didn't even know she was having her period. I used to think, 'Why can't I be like that?'"

When Eve got to school, she sat at her desk with the heels of her feet on her chair and her knees pressed against her chest, an attempt to find a position comfortable enough that she could try to concentrate on the lesson being taught. When she got home, she lay on her bed in a fetal position, unable to move. Sometimes she even enlisted the help of her dog. "I'd have my dog lie on my stomach. The heat and pressure from the dog would sometimes make the pain subside a little bit."

As soon as she was old enough to go to the doctor without her mom, she did. "I went to the doctor and he said this was normal. I said, 'This is normal? There is no way this is normal!' But he wouldn't listen." She didn't know where else to turn, so she silently suffered for years. As she got older, she continued to try to find a comfortable position in which to sit or lie down, but instead of a school desk, she was sitting at her work desk, and instead of her dog lying on top of her, she pressed multiple heating pads against her body.

Eve also took multiple pain medications, and in heavy doses. It was like throwing a small cup of water on a raging inferno. "I was like a pregnant woman going through contractions that never stopped," she said. "Then the pain expanded into my bowel area to the point that I felt like my bowels were going to explode. It was a very emotional time. I was just a mess."

Cramps are normal. Killer cramps are not normal. Every woman with endometriosis will try to convince herself that what she is feeling is the way it's supposed to be, especially if other people, including doctors, are telling her that. She won't slow down. She won't give in to the pain. But remember, the pain you are feeling is real, no matter what anybody else tries to tell you. It is your brain telling you that something is wrong. If the pain is excessive, then listen to it. Don't fight it, because you won't win.

8

Painful Sex

THE THIRD CARDINAL SYMPTOM OF endometriosis is painful sex. Heavy periods are personal. Killer cramps are personal. But painful sex is about as personal and private as it gets. For a woman to have to talk openly with anybody, even those close to her, about the physical challenges she experiences with intercourse is extremely difficult. When a woman visits my office for the first time and tells me her symptoms, it's rare for her to voluntarily mention painful sex as being one of them. I usually have to ask her multiple times if it's an issue before she will admit that it is. It's an important fact for me to know because it can help me determine her level of pain and where in her body the endometriosis is located. And it's an important fact for her to disclose, not only for the good of her physical health, but also because the symptom is one that can cause tension in, or even break up, a relationship.

How does endometriosis cause pain during sex? As discussed in an earlier chapter, the area behind the uterus is called the cul-de-sac, or pouch of Douglas. Normally it is lined by smooth peritoneum, the skin-like sheet of tissue that covers the uterus and vagina anteriorly (in front) and the rectum posteriorly (in back), keeping the rectum, vagina, and uterus free from each other. Endometriosis will frequently adhere the vagina to the rectum. The pain caused by endometriosis during intercourse is deep; it comes from the inflammation and fibrosis fusing the front wall of the rectum to the back wall of the vagina. Mobility and expansion of the upper posterior vagina behind the cervix normally occurs during sex, but not if endometriosis is present. The pain can be more intense in certain sexual positions than in others, depending on exactly where the endometriosis is located and how advanced it is. If it's widespread, the woman may hurt no matter what position she's in.

A woman experiencing pain during intercourse often will not complain about it. She will tolerate it to a high degree perhaps because she doesn't want to interrupt the intimacy. She might be afraid of rejection, or loves her partner too much to let anything stand between them. To her, the emotional side of sex, the intimacy, trumps the physical pain she has to endure. Sometimes a woman will even subconsciously refuse to accept that sex is painful because she fears how her partner will react. She doesn't want to be accused of not returning love or intimacy, or of having no interest in her partner, so she convinces herself that everything is fine.

From her partner's perspective, it is difficult to know what the woman is going through because of how well she covers up her pain during intercourse. At worst, her partner may assume that sex is a little uncomfortable for her, but that it's nothing to be concerned about because *she* is not expressing concern. Even a couple who has had a strong relationship for several years can face struggles if the disease causes the frequency of sex to diminish. I have seen this happen often. It's another reason why diagnosing and treating endometriosis early is so important. Nobody wants it to reach a stage in which it is affecting the patient's intimate relationship.

One of my patients, Beth, was eleven years old when she had her first period, and it was an extremely painful one. "I was at school when it happened, and I came home crying because I had never experienced pain like that in my life," she said. "Every month from then on I experienced excruciating pain for three or four days. I grew up on a military base, so I went to the hospital there and they said, 'You're a female; this is normal.' It continued to be really bad for about the next five years. When I turned sixteen and would have my periods, I would curl up in a ball and sometimes pass out. They started me on birth control, but that didn't do anything. Neither did ibuprofen. When I went to college, I just assumed that I would have to shut down during my period. I would have to plan my life around those three to five days every month."

Her first sexual experience was with her college boyfriend when she was nineteen. "It was horrible," she said. "I just thought maybe I didn't like it because it hurt. It was not as painful as my menstrual cramps, but it was very uncomfortable. It didn't feel right. It didn't feel normal. I also started to notice that my checkups with my OB/GYN were incredibly painful. The doctor would just say, 'What's wrong? Relax. This shouldn't hurt.' It made me very scared to go to the doctor each year."

Beth, now thirty-two, is married. She and her husband dated for six years before they were engaged, so they'd been together for a while before I diagnosed her with endometriosis and did surgery on her in 2012. The endometriosis impacted their sex life during the years before surgery. Her husband knew intercourse caused her pain. She said sometimes they would go for a couple of months without being intimate. "It wasn't easy, that's for sure," Beth said. But their deep emotional love for one another helped them both get through their struggles.

"I loved him so much that I wanted to be close to him physically. I wanted that for us more than I cared about my own comfort," Beth said. "At the same time, he was very respectful and careful with me. He knew it was a physical issue, and he was very understanding. If sex had been the most important thing to him, then our relationship wouldn't have made it. That intimacy is important in a relationship, so it was frustrating when it couldn't happen as often as we wanted, but we are so interested in each other mentally. It's not easy, but you can definitely overcome it when the love is there."

NOTE: See image 17 in the photo section starting on page 93.

9

Cut with Razor Blades

THE FOURTH CARDINAL SYMPTOM OF endometriosis is painful bowel movements. A bowel movement is when your stool passes through and out of your body after the food you've eaten has gone through your digestive tract. What needs to be understood about this symptom is the off-the-charts level of pain that can come with it. We've all had painful bowel movements, but painful bowel movements caused by endometriosis are a completely different story. Painful bowel movements, along with symptoms of constipation during menstruation or pain during sex, are significant signs that endometriosis is located in the large bowel.

I did a five-and-a-half-hour surgery on a patient named Monique in 2015, and her insides were a mess. I removed endometriosis, fibroids, her appendix, part of her small intestine, an ovary, and a fallopian tube. One of the many symptoms of endometriosis that she had going into surgery was painful bowel movements.

"When I went to the bathroom to move my bowels, it wasn't a pain issue with straining, like a lot of people feel. It literally felt like my insides were being cut with razor blades as the feces moved through," she said.

Monique said she finally realized after a few months that the bowel pain was only there during her menstruation cycle. She shared that information with her OB/GYN. "When I told her, she just kind of said, 'Okay. Uh-huh.' She never addressed it. She never said it could be this or that. She never asked me any questions about it. I had just told her that it felt like I was passing razor blades—it was that painful—and she showed no concern at all."

Like painful sex, it's never easy for someone to talk about something as personal as her bowels. What disturbs me the most about Monique's story is that even though she knew something was wrong inside her, and even though she had the courage to tell her doctor about this very personal symptom, she was rebuffed and told that it was no big deal. Doctors can easily recognize endometriosis that involves the appendix. But experienced gynecologic surgeons, as well as general surgeons, often miss endometriosis of the intestines, such as the rectum and sigmoid. Even gastroenterologists almost always miss endometriosis located in the bowel during a colonoscopy. We all occasionally have painful bowels, but few of us describe the sensation as feeling like we are passing razor blades. If you have that symptom along with constipation, especially during your period, and you get nothing more than an "okay" or an "uh-huh" from your doctor, find another doctor, and make sure your new one considers endometriosis as a possible diagnosis.

10

Neuropathy

THE FIFTH CARDINAL SYMPTOM, NEUROPATHY, is pain caused by damaged nerves. When you have neuropathy, the nerves are physically attacked, directly or indirectly, by the endometriosis. It could be scar tissue pulling the nerve, or the disease attacking the nerve. Pain from neuropathy caused by endometriosis will generally be felt in the back, leg (sciatica), or crotch area. The sharper the pain, the more likely it is that a lesion is pushing directly on a nerve.

You read about neuropathy in Lauren's story. Her pain was widespread, affecting even her back and legs. With much difficulty I was able to remove a lot of diseased tissue around her nerves, especially from those in the deep pelvic sidewalls affecting her legs. "The pain in my legs, lower back, sides, and hips was always there to go with all the other pain I had," Lauren said. "Before the surgery, I had a lot of trouble walking. It's funny to think about it now, but I kind of waddled like a duck—that's how much it hurt. I couldn't walk straight no matter how hard I tried. It was a very throbbing, constant, stabbing pain, especially when I was very active."

In 2011, soon after her second laser surgery with another doctor, Annie Rose experienced so much pain in her left leg that she could barely walk. She called the doctor and told him it felt as if she were being stung by a thousand bees at once, and she was certain the endometriosis had spread into her leg. "He told me that was impossible," Annie Rose said.

"He told me that he'd gotten it all, and that it couldn't be in my leg because endometriosis doesn't leave the pelvic area. But I had read about it and knew that wasn't true. Now I couldn't even trust my own doctor." Soon afterward, she was in an elevator at work and collapsed. Her legs hurt so badly that they gave out on her. She eventually lost nearly all mobility in her left leg. "I had to physically move it with my arms to get it to work," she said.

Jessica, who believes that endometriosis "proves how physically and mentally strong you really are," endured leg pain so severe in college that she had difficulty getting out of bed to go to class. She underwent several unsuccessful laser surgeries before she found me in 2012. I performed deep-excision surgery on her after finding a widespread case of endometriosis that affected the nerves in her legs, which was why she struggled to walk.

These and other stories about neuropathy from my patients could also be recorded in the "Misdiagnoses" section of this book. Neuropathy is a significant symptom of endometriosis, but it is often mistaken by doctors as a symptom of something completely unrelated to the disease.

Elisa, a patient from Staten Island, suffered horrible leg pain for several months. Her sciatic nerve, which extends into the leg, was being compressed in her pelvis by endometriosis. Her doctor was unfamiliar with endometriosis, however, so it was never considered as a source of the pain. "I thought it was tendinitis because that's what my doctor thought it was," Elisa said. "I was put in a boot, but that didn't help. Then I went through acupuncture and physical therapy, but neither helped."

Like all symptoms, neuropathy alone is not a sign of endometriosis. But something such as leg pain combined with other symptoms that worsen with menstruation could mean that endometriosis is affecting your leg and is messing with your nerves. If you have any or all of the classic symptoms of endometriosis, and then neuropathy kicks in, get it treated before further damage is done. A cold is just a cold until it is ignored or misdiagnosed; then it can turn into bronchitis or a sinus infection or pneumonia. It's no different with endometriosis, or any other disease for that matter. The more time that goes by before it is treated, the more it can spread throughout your body, and the more long-term health complications it can cause.

11

Four Miscarriages...
and a Baby

ENDOMETRIOSIS IS THE ONE DISEASE with which fertility problems are most closely associated. Many times, a woman who has difficulty conceiving will have a case of endometriosis that does not come with severe symptoms. This is known as *silent endometriosis*. These silent sufferers eagerly crowd into the waiting rooms of in vitro fertilization (IVF) clinics with the hope of conceiving. IVF is a method in which a woman's eggs are collected and fertilized by sperm in a lab, then implanted in her uterus. These women are often not told they may have endometriosis, and the in vitro attempts they take will generally fail. If these patients question the possibility of endometriosis as the cause for the failure, they are usually falsely assured by their fertility specialist that endometriosis does not have a negative, or even significant, impact in conception. Sometimes, they will even claim that pregnancy will cure a patient's endometriosis. By the time multiple IVF attempts have failed, these patients, at this point between thirty-five and forty years old, are told that their ovaries have no reserves left and that egg quality is poor.

But when endometriosis is removed by excision surgery, inflammatory tissue from the ovary and around the fallopian tubes is also removed. As a result, patients may not only increase their rate of success with IVF, but also, not infrequently, get pregnant naturally without assisted technologies. I mentioned that the American Society for Reproductive

Medicine says endometriosis can be found in up to 50 percent of infertile women. People are often shocked by that statistic since endometriosis is still unfamiliar to many, but it is nonetheless true.

Many patients who were unable to get pregnant when they first came to me—even those with stage III or IV endometriosis—got pregnant following deep-excision surgery because all abnormal endometriosis tissue was removed and pelvic organs were restored to their normal state. Endometriosis does not *directly* cause infertility, but patients who have the disease will have a significantly lower chance of getting pregnant. Why? The first reason concerns the unfriendly molecules produced by the inflammation of endometriosis. These molecules (cytokines) have a paralyzing effect on the sperm and the egg and prevent the fertilization process. The second reason is that endometriosis physically distorts a woman's pelvic anatomy. Again, the inflammatory process changes the fine transparent texture of the peritoneum. It produces scarring and adhesions, which can cause the fallopian tubes and ovaries to become blocked, preventing the sperm and egg from coming into contact with each other. Further, the ovaries may fail to ovulate, causing eggs to become trapped in the ovaries. All these obstacles in a woman's reproductive system can prevent pregnancy or cause very complicated pregnancies, including miscarriages.

The case of Michele, a patient of mine, is a perfect example of the link between endometriosis and infertility. She was about sixteen years old when she started to experience some of the symptoms of the disease. In the late 1980s, when she was twenty-two and the pain was increasing, a sonogram showed that she had a small ovarian cyst. Her doctor tried to shrink it by prescribing birth control pills, but that didn't work. Six weeks later, the cyst ruptured. Her doctor performed emergency surgery and was able to save the ovary, but she noticed during surgery that Michele had endometriosis. The only option she gave Michele for treating it was a hysterectomy. Michele hadn't had any children yet and wasn't ready to have any of her reproductive organs removed. Over roughly the next decade, two more cysts developed on the same ovary at separate times. Both were removed by a different doctor (her previous doctor had retired), who also told her that a hysterectomy was the only way to treat the endometriosis.

"I had just gotten married two years before the last cyst was removed, and my doctor said that if I wanted to have a baby, I really should try then before things got worse and I wouldn't be able to have kids at all," Michele said. So she tried to get pregnant and did, but the pregnancy ended in a miscarriage. This happened two more times.

"It was a really dark time in my life," Michele said, fighting back tears more than fifteen years later. "But I was determined. I didn't want to give up. I felt it was a positive thing that I was able to get pregnant, but why wasn't I able to carry the baby full term? I eventually learned that the endometriosis played a big role in that."

When another cyst developed after the third miscarriage, Michele was determined to find a doctor who specialized in endometriosis. Through the Internet (a fairly new phenomenon back then), she found a doctor in Oregon who referred her to a doctor closer to her New York City home: my mentor, Dr. Harry Reich. "My organs were all stuck together," Michele said. "Dr. Reich operated on me for six hours and afterward told me that the endometriosis had been blocking my tubes. He didn't say I could have a child—nobody can promise that—but he said he gave it his best shot and removed 99 percent of the endometriosis."

In 2000, Michele was pregnant again, this time with twins. "The pregnancy was an emotional roller coaster," she said. "I lost one of the babies after four months." But the other one survived.

"I was so grateful that I was able to have him," she said. "When I gave birth, it was a horrible experience. I was induced and in so much pain. The epidural didn't work, my blood pressure dropped. I pushed him out in, like, twenty minutes, but then they took him from me because he was having breathing problems. He stayed in NICU [neonatal intensive care unit] for four days. It was so nerve-wracking. But everything turned out fine. I had my baby, and he has grown up into a healthy kid."

Three years later Michele had the daughter she'd always wanted. "And thankfully it was a very uneventful pregnancy and birth," she said.

Michele's endometriosis returned nearly a decade after Dr. Reich had done surgery on her. He was retiring, so she came to me. I removed the disease, but six years later it was back yet again. She finally decided a hysterectomy was in order, two children and nearly twenty-six years after she was told by her first doctor that a hysterectomy was her only option. "I know my surgery with Dr. Reich is why I was able to have kids at all," Michele said. "I could have had the hysterectomy so much sooner, but I just wasn't ready."

I will discuss hysterectomies in the sections on misdiagnoses and on alternative treatments. I shared Michele's story with you now to get across two very important points about infertility. One is that endometriosis can, and often does, prevent a woman from getting pregnant. If you are trying to get pregnant but can't, and if you have other symptoms of the disease, consider the possibility that you have endometriosis. The other point is that deep-excision surgery can reverse infertility problems. No doctor can guarantee anything, as Michele said. But deep-excision surgery can give you hope, including the hope of having children.

12

Fatigue

WHEN DISCUSSING THE PHYSICAL EFFECTS of endometriosis, pain is generally the main symptom doctors focus on, as they should. It's the one thing that all women with this disease have in common in some form. But coming in a close second is fatigue. The main cause of endometriosis-related fatigue is the body's effort to eliminate the diseased tissue. While the immune system attempts to combat endometriosis, cytokines, also known as inflammatory toxins, are secreted by the tissue. What patients feel to be fatigue is the result of these internal chemicals. Many women and their doctors lump fatigue together with pain, but the two are very different monsters. Fatigue is a constant state of being tired—not sleepy, but physically exhausted. Though pain can accompany fatigue, or even be a primary cause of it, you don't necessarily hurt when you feel fatigue. Your body just says, "I'm done. I have no energy to do anything."

One reason why women with endometriosis-related fatigue don't discuss it much is that, as is the case with many endometriosis symptoms, a stigma surrounds it. When you say you're in pain people normally listen to you and show some concern, even if they don't know you have endometriosis, don't understand why you are in pain, and don't know what to do about it. But when you say you're too tired to do something, people often consider you lazy or out of shape, or they may take your rejection personally, especially if they know you didn't exert a lot of energy that day and have, in their ill-informed opinion, no valid reason for being so tired.

Before surgery, Annie Rose suffered an extreme amount of pain, but fatigue debilitated her even more. She went to work, returned home, lay down on the couch, and was out of commission until she had to do it over again the next morning. Annie Rose is one of the hardest-working women I know. She went years without taking a sick day at work despite the constant agony inflicted on her by endometriosis. Still, friends who wanted her to go out with them questioned the validity of her claims that she was too tired.

"It's a different kind of tired," Annie Rose said. "You feel like you're being tranquilized, like something has taken over your body. My eyes would get heavy and swollen. I couldn't do anything. And when I felt that level of fatigue, it was a warning sign that a flare-up of pain from the endometriosis was coming."

Liza, the patient who stated that she was never asked by her previous doctor about the painful periods she noted on her paperwork, is one of the few patients I've had who felt more fatigue than pain. I've said that the level of pain a woman feels does not necessarily reflect how widespread the endometriosis is. Liza is a perfect example of that. I performed a four-and-a-half-hour surgery on her and removed twenty-seven tissue specimens, twenty-six of which tested positive for endometriosis. Yet during the ten-plus years that she went undiagnosed she reported much less pain than most women. She had silent endometriosis. But the fatigue hit her hard beginning in her early twenties.

"I would come home and just collapse. It was utter exhaustion," Liza said. "Most weekends I didn't want to do anything. When I told doctors about it, they would say that I was too stressed or that I wasn't eating enough. It didn't make sense. I exercised and ate well all the time." The fatigue lasted into her early thirties until I excised the endometriosis in 2015. "Now I definitely have more energy; it's wonderful," she said. "But it was very difficult before that. I think people just assume that everybody is tired because we all live hectic lives in this country, but this was very different."

Annie Rose implores women who experience deep fatigue to listen to their bodies, just as they do when they feel pain. She also wants friends, family members, and coworkers of endometriosis patients to understand that there is a legitimate reason why the patients feel the way they do.

"I went from being a bubbly, enthusiastic person who was full of life all the time to being someone hit so hard by fatigue that I became a lifeless person just lying there," she said. "I didn't want to be that way. People need to try to understand that there was a reason for it. I know that may be difficult because they've never gone through it themselves, but it's very real."

13

Genetics

A YOUNG WOMAN WHO HAS a mother or sister with endometriosis is about six times more likely to develop it herself. Genetics plays a major role in the disease. Many of my patients tell me they have the same symptoms their mothers once had, such as killer cramps and painful periods that began at a very young age. Most say their mothers tolerated the pain and expected their daughters to do the same. In some cases the mothers underwent hysterectomies but never explained to their daughters why. My guess is the mothers may not have known exactly why themselves. Their doctors probably recommended a hysterectomy as a remedy for the pain they were experiencing, but without diagnosing endometriosis as the source of the pain.

As you read earlier, Padma learned that her mother had endured the same painful symptoms Padma experienced. You also read that Lauren's mother had the disease, but neither Lauren nor her mother thought there could be a genetic link. "My mom feels bad about it today," Lauren said. "She says, 'I gave you this horrible disease.' But I tell her she shouldn't feel that way. I joke with her that I have been fighting this disease since I was an embryo. There is nothing she could have done about it."

Elisa, the patient with neuropathy who was told by her doctor that it was tendinitis, sent her sister to see me because her sister had symptoms similar to those of Elisa. Sure enough, her sister also had the disease.

Eve, who said that her mother never felt pain with her periods, is pretty certain her grandmother did. "My grandmother had a hysterectomy, but she never told anybody why," Eve said. "I believe now that endometriosis may have been the reason why. It was in the late 1920s. She never told my mother that maybe she should watch for problems that I might have one day. My grandmother always kept things hush-hush."

Monique, who felt like her insides were being cut with razor blades during bowel movements, said her mother had fibroids and a full hysterectomy at age thirty-six. Monique also had fibroids in addition to her endometriosis. She was encouraged multiple times by previous doctors to have a hysterectomy when she was in her thirties.

That's five women out of about a dozen you have met so far who had a mother, sister, or grandmother who also had or may have had endometriosis. These women were selected for this book because of the impact of their stories, not because there may have been genetic links with their disease. For nearly half of them to have a possible genetic connection is significant. Many of my patients with endometriosis who became mothers expressed enormous concern about their daughters potentially inheriting the same disease. And they have valid reasons to be concerned.

The ROSE Project, which my foundation helped start, is committed to finding a genetic link to, and eventually a nonsurgical cure for, endometriosis. (More about the ROSE Project appears later.) Today, what is important for you to know is that if your mother or sister or grandmother was diagnosed with the disease, or if she was not diagnosed but had the symptoms, you stand a greater chance of having it. That's why including education in efforts to combat endometriosis is so important—why an adolescent girl, for example, needs to know what is normal and what is not normal once her menstrual cycle beings. It is also one more reason why there has been a concerted effort in recent years for women and men to know the history of health in their families. Much of that effort has revolved around cancer and heart disease, but health education should include everything, even endometriosis.

Misdiagnoses

14

"It Was All So Stupid"

MANY PEOPLE WOULD AGREE THAT receiving the wrong diagnosis from a doctor is worse than receiving no diagnosis at all. Of course, neither is a good thing. Getting no diagnosis is certainly frustrating, but a misdiagnosis can put a patient on a path that leads her further away from determining what is really wrong. It can result in her being prescribed medication that does nothing to fix the real problem and could have detrimental side effects. It can cost her valuable time in finding the real cause of her symptoms because she stops looking. It can also cause her to lose trust in her doctor, and possibly doctors in general.

Most of my patients were misdiagnosed by other doctors at least once and often multiple times. What they were told ranged from "You have irritable bowel syndrome" to "It's all in your head." The doctors lacked the experience to know what the real problem was. Some of them didn't even give their patients the sense that they really cared about them, especially if they discounted their pain as not being real. To cap it off, some of the remedies they recommended were downright crazy.

Stephanie, a patient from northern New Jersey, suffered with endometriosis pain for roughly fifteen years, during which time she was misdiagnosed several times. Her gut told her that there was something gynecologically wrong with her, but she could not find a doctor to agree, so she put her faith in their inaccurate assessments. That faith cost her a lot of time, along with her uterus and both ovaries. When she came to me in 2015, I operated on her for several hours, removing eighteen lesions from her pelvis. Today, she is pain-free and feels like a new woman at age forty-five. But she is still bothered by the fact that it took so long to get the proper diagnosis. While she knew that the responsibility lay primarily on her doctors' shoulders, she blamed herself—until she read the testimonials of some of my patients.

"To be honest, I felt stupid for listening to those doctors," Stephanie said. "But then I read what the other women wrote, how similar their stories were to mine, and I said, 'Oh my gosh, it's not just me. There are other women who have this.' "

Stephanie didn't experience endometriosis symptoms at a young age, the way many of my patients did. She had three children without any complications. But sometime between giving birth to her second and third children, around age thirty, she felt pain on the left side of her pelvic area during her period. She went to her gynecologist, who told her that she had a small cyst on her left ovary.

"He said it was no big deal," Stephanie said. "But then the pain got worse. I had a hard time sleeping and had to ask my mom to help me with the kids. I didn't understand what was going on because I had never felt that pain before. I went back to my OB/GYN, and he told me again that I was fine. He sent me back to my regular doctor." Stephanie told her doctor that she and her husband were trying to get pregnant and were in the process of moving out of state.

"He said the pain was probably from the stress of those two things," she said. "Being in my thirties and having never experienced pain like that before, I just accepted what he said. I figured it certainly was possible that it was stress."

As time went on, the pain intensified and spread to her right side. She returned to her doctor, who told her she should—brace yourself— see a therapist. "I thought it was completely ridiculous, but I didn't know what else to do," Stephanie said. "I thought that if this was what was wrong with me, then it's what I needed to do. I trusted him." Stephanie went to a few sessions. She was told to try yoga and to practice breathing techniques using her stomach. The therapist also wanted to talk about her past. "We talked about my family. I told her we moved around a lot when I was a kid. She tried to say that maybe my pain had something to do with post-traumatic stress from all that moving. It was all so stupid. That pain was in my pelvis, not in my head, and the only thing that was going to get rid of it was for someone to go in and physically remove it."

The pain continued to spread, this time to her lower back. A new doctor told her it was probably triggered by her picking up her kids too much. When she got pregnant with her third child, the pain subsided considerably. (Pregnancy sometimes alleviates a woman's endometriosis pain because she doesn't have her periods when she is pregnant.) But in the months after she gave birth, it returned. "I didn't even tell my doctor because I didn't want to be told again that it was stress," she said. The pain became so severe that she finally went to see her gynecologist. He told her she had another cyst on her left ovary.

"I was like, 'Really? That's it? I think there is something more going on.'" But he told her he couldn't find anything else wrong. She went to another doctor, who prescribed a drug designed to treat panic and anxiety disorders. It provided no relief. She went back to her gynecologist, who sent her to get an MRI. It revealed the cyst on her left ovary and a possible tumor on her appendix. The doctor also thought she may have needed her colon resected. He wanted to do surgery. Thinking this might solve her issues, since the diagnosis was physical and different from anything else she'd been diagnosed with, and since the tumor on her appendix seemed like a legitimate source of pain, Stephanie agreed to the surgery.

"When I woke up, they said the tumor was benign, and they didn't have to touch my colon. But they said I had endometriosis everywhere: on the bladder, the cul-de-sac, the peritoneal lining. There was also significant scarring on my left side where the pain had originated so many years earlier. For the first time, it all made sense," she said. "I was in my forties, had all those issues, and never had any idea what was wrong. Now, suddenly, I knew. It was unbelievable."

Soon after Stephanie's surgery, she saw a television ad looking for women to participate in an endometriosis study. A woman in the commercial was shown with barbed wire wrapped tightly around her waist. "That's exactly what the pain always felt like to me," she said. "I was baffled that none of my doctors had asked me if that's what the pain was like."

Even though she now had a diagnosis, she still wasn't in the clear. After the surgery, her surgeon sent her back to her gynecologist, who put her on Lupron, a drug that sends a woman into menopause to stop her periods (I will talk more about Lupron later). "It was awful, awful, awful. I was on a dose that required me to take a shot every three months. I was a mess. My blood pressure shot through the roof."

She switched to a new OB/GYN, a woman who Stephanie thought might understand her better. The doctor suggested a hysterectomy to remove the uterus and both ovaries. As I will discuss later, a hysterectomy is often suggested by doctors who don't know how to properly treat endometriosis. When I do surgery, removing any organ, especially a reproductive one, is my absolute last resort. But not knowing where else to turn, Stephanie agreed. When she woke up after surgery, the doctor told her she'd removed the uterus and ovaries, but hadn't taken out any of the endometriosis that was stuck to the other organs because she was afraid of damaging the organs.

"I felt marginally better," Stephanie said. "She told me the disease would dry up in about six weeks because the ovaries were out." Since estrogen and progesterone were no longer being produced to feed the endometriosis, the doctor theorized that the endometriosis tissue clinging to the other organs would disappear. It didn't. Stephanie's pain soon returned in full force. That's when she finally found me. She'd read a story in *People* magazine about Padma's battle with endometriosis. Stephanie did not want to undergo another surgery, but she felt confident after our first meeting that I would be able to take care of her the way she should have been taken care of fifteen years earlier.

One of the last things Stephanie asked her OB/GYN before finding me was if she should worry about her teenage daughter getting the disease. "She said I shouldn't even tell her about it because there was no reason to worry her," Stephanie said. "But when I went to Dr. Seckin, he asked if I had a daughter, asked what her periods were like, and suggested that I bring her in for a checkup. My OB/GYN was a female, yet she was telling me to keep this quiet from my daughter. She was so misinformed."

As long as doctors remain misinformed about endometriosis, patients will be misdiagnosed. They will continue to suffer unnecessarily, and they will be treated for conditions they don't have while the disease progresses in their bodies.

The chapters in this section will identify some of the most common misdiagnoses for endometriosis, including irritable bowel syndrome and appendicitis. Other diseases for which endometriosis is sometimes mistaken include sexually transmitted diseases, fibroids, diverticulitis, pelvic inflammatory disease, colon cancer, and ovarian cancer. Understand these misdiagnoses, and learn about others. As you read in Stephanie's account, doctors can concoct some pretty wild things—not on purpose, but because they don't have the knowledge or experience necessary to diagnose endometriosis. If a doctor can tell a woman with endometriosis that her pelvic pain may be traceable to the number of times she moved as a child, then seemingly anything is possible. Trust your doctor, but trust yourself and your pain more. You must be your own advocate. If your doctor's diagnosis doesn't seem right to you, then you are the one who is probably right.

NOTE: See image 13 in the photo section starting on page 93.

15

IBS: A Dump Diagnosis

IRRITABLE BOWEL SYNDROME, OR IBS, is a relatively common disorder that affects the colon. Many of its symptoms are similar to those of endometriosis, such as diarrhea, constipation, bloating, cramping, and abdominal pain. Unlike endometriosis, IBS can be more or less controlled with medication or a change in diet. Surgery is rarely needed. Doctors often mistake endometriosis for IBS because of the similarities in symptoms and because they don't know much, if anything, about endometriosis. I know that the intentions of these doctors are very good—they want their patients to get well—but their knowledge is limited.

The doctor, usually a gastroenterologist, will begin his or her investigative process by viewing the upper gastrointestinal tract through a scope inserted through the patient's mouth, down the esophagus, and into the stomach. The doctor will then insert a scope through her anus to check her rectum and colon. If all findings are perfectly normal, the doctor will often conclude that she has IBS, without noticing the inflammation in the outer layer of the bowels. It's what I call a *dump diagnosis:* a go-to diagnosis when the doctor doesn't know what else it could be. It's similar to Freud's diagnosing women with hysteria more than a century ago. More of my patients than I can count have been erroneously diagnosed with IBS at some stage in their battle with endometriosis.

What do these doctors fail to ask the patient that could help reveal what she is really battling? The magic question: *Do the symptoms of consti-pation, painful bowel movements, or diarrhea occur at the same time as your period?* Again, they don't ask because they don't know why to ask.

When the doctor is evaluating the patient—looking into the stom-ach, the colon, the rectum—he or she is looking *inside* those organs for a potential source of the pain, not on the *outside.* Nor does the doctor refer the patient to someone who can look on the outside if he or she is not equipped or skilled to do so. So what do they recommend as a solution to their patient's supposed illness? They typically have her make some dietary adjustments, which may temporarily calm the bowel symptoms, giving the false impression that the problem is fixed. But the symptoms inevitably return, and usually very quickly.

A classic case of an IBS misdiagnosis involved Elisa, the patient whose leg pain was incorrectly diagnosed as tendinitis. Elisa was diagnosed with endometriosis at age thirty-three. I would guess, based on what she told me about her health history, that she'd probably had the disease since she was twelve. I am certain she had it by the time she was seventeen, when she was in the bathroom with diarrhea quite often during very heavy periods.

"They did five endoscopies [to check the digestive tract] in the years after that, and they did two colonoscopies," Elisa said. "They really couldn't tell for sure what I had, so they told me it was IBS. The prob-lem was that they were looking on the inside of my organs and not the outside." Their fix was to give Elisa fluids through an IV to keep her hydrated and to put her on a special diet that included foods low in acid. "It didn't improve my health because I didn't have IBS," she said.

Between ages seventeen and twenty-one, Elisa passed out five times from severe abdominal pain. "I saw different OB/GYNs, and none of them picked up on the endometriosis," she said. "I should have been diagnosed with it when I was seventeen. It's amazing that all those years they thought I had something that I never had."

Annie Rose was misdiagnosed with IBS in the early 2000s, at about age twenty-five, after a gastroenterologist did a colonoscopy on her. "I was having some bowel issues, and my mom recommended that I see him. I was feeling bloated, gassy, and experienced constant pressure," she said. "He told me that I had IBS and internal hemorrhoids, and that was it. There was really no follow-through. No meds or any special diet. He just said to try to eat more watermelon and deal with the pain. I felt if he wasn't going to make a big deal out of it, then I wasn't going to make a big deal out of it. Unfortunately, I never made the connection between my bowel issue and my period, and he never asked."

I want to be very clear that if you are a woman diagnosed with IBS, you should not assume it's a misdiagnosis. You may very well have the condition, and if you do, a gastroenterologist will certainly know how to treat it. But if your doctor's treatment isn't working, or if your pain or other symptoms occur each month during your period, understand that what you have may be much more than IBS—and do your best to make your doctor understand that, too. That is one of the primary purposes of this book: to educate you about endometriosis so that you can both be your own advocate and also bring any necessary awareness to your doctor, who may have little or no knowledge of the disease.

Elisa was at a disadvantage because she had never heard of endometriosis when she was diagnosed with IBS as a teenager in the 1990s. In fact, Elisa is a nurse who was never taught about endometriosis in nursing school. If you are misdiagnosed with IBS when what you truly have is endometriosis, the misdiagnosis gives the endometriosis more time to grow, which can create more problems and significantly more risk as time progresses. Don't stop listening to your body after you see your doctor. Pay attention to how your body reacts to the treatment you receive, and speak up if it's not working.

16

Hysterectomy Bad

I'M GOING TO SHARE SOME extremely important information about hysterectomies, and I will support that information with two horrifying stories: one from Monique, whom you've already met, and one from Julie, a patient of mine who had a hysterectomy by another doctor when she was still a teenager. If your doctor ever suggests that you should have a hysterectomy to relieve your endometriosis pain (or pain caused by anything else), your brain should go on high alert. There are occasions when a hysterectomy may be necessary, but often it is not, even though your doctor may try to convince you that there are no other options.

A hysterectomy is the removal of the uterus (womb). It can also include the removal of the ovaries, fallopian tubes, and cervix. Once the uterus is taken out, it cannot be put back in, and a woman can no longer have children. That's why it can be such an emotionally difficult surgery for a woman to undergo. Having a hysterectomy isn't always a bad thing (see the chapter titled "Hysterectomy Not So Bad"), but it *must be an absolute last resort* for treating endometriosis, especially in women who still want to have children or think they may want to. Unfortunately, many doctors who aren't well versed in endometriosis, especially those who do not know how to do deep-excision surgery (or who are unfamiliar with the procedure), don't think that way. They may tell their patients that the only solution to their ailment is to remove their uterus.

A hysterectomy is usually needed when there is evidence of adeno-myosis—when endometriosis cells develop in the muscle tissue of the uterus. It is often called a "sister" disease to endometriosis. Like endome-triosis, there is no way to prevent adenomyosis. Its most common symp-toms are severe pain and heavy periods. As one can imagine, the pain is excruciating-times-two for a woman who has both adenomyosis within the wall of her uterus and endometriosis implants on the outside. In the absence of adenomyosis, a hysterectomy is a "quick fix" that likely won't fix anything, and it can actually make matters psychologically worse for a woman who has just lost any chance of ever carrying a child.

A hysterectomy is a procedure, not a misdiagnosis. I've nonetheless included this chapter because many doctors perform hysterectomies as their treatment for what is usually a misdiagnosis. I want to drive home the point that if your doctor tells you a hysterectomy is your only solu-tion, you need to be skeptical. I'm not saying your doctor is wrong. I'm saying you must question him or her, and you must not hesitate to seek multiple opinions.

You need to understand, and you need to do your best to make your doctor(s) understand, that if you have endometriosis, removing the uter-us does nothing more than that: it removes that one organ, but it does not address other regions where the endometriosis may remain. In other words, the pain will still likely be there after the uterus is removed, and the disease will continue to spread, so nothing is accomplished.

Yes, your doctor could be correct; removing your uterus may be the right solution, but you need to find out first why deep-excision surgery is not a better solution. If your doctor says, "What's that?" or if he or she doesn't do that kind of surgery, you need to get another opinion . . . or two . . . or three . . . or four, as Monique did.

Monique didn't start having painful periods until 2008, when she was in her midthirties. She described her cycles as "horrific"—painful periods, nausea, painful urination, painful bowel movements. "I went to my gynecologist, and she said everything was fine," Monique said. "I told her my periods hurt and that sometimes my uterus hurt even when I wasn't having my period. She said it was no big deal, so I just assumed it was part of getting older."

In 2012, Monique's doctor spotted what looked like a cyst on her right ovary. "She wasn't sure what it was, so she sent me to a specialist. His bedside manner was horrible," Monique said. "He asked me a couple of questions, including whether or not I wanted to get pregnant, because he thought I should have a hysterectomy. I said that I would like to have a child one day, but even if I don't or can't, I don't want to be cut up unnecessarily. He said he wasn't sure how else to deal with the cyst, so he sent me to another doctor, who also said I needed a hysterectomy. I said, 'Wait a minute. How did I go from a cyst to a hysterectomy?' But nobody told me anything. They didn't even tell me what caused the cyst." Monique decided to live with the pain the best she could; she was not ready to have a hysterectomy.

Over the next couple of years, the pain worsened. She had to go to the emergency room a couple of times. She was given Lupron to put her into early menopause. She had a cyst drained, giving her temporary relief, but the cyst was still there. She was shuffled from doctor to doctor. In fact, a third doctor recommended that she have a hysterectomy, which she continued to refuse to do. "Through all this, nobody mentioned endometriosis to me," Monique said. "They did rule out cancer, but that was all they could tell me. I had no idea what was going on."

In 2014, Monique went back to her original gynecologist, who said endometrial cells were found in the fluid that was drained from the cyst. It was the first time endometriosis had been discussed. Monique took control of her situation from there. "I googled 'endometriosis specialist,'" which is how she found me.

When she came into my office for her first visit and I diagnosed her with endometriosis, she told me about her wish to keep her organs, which I respected. I couldn't make her any promises, as I never can, but I told her I would try my best because I knew how important that was to her. The surgery lasted nearly six hours. For the good of her overall health, I had no choice but to remove her appendix, part of her small intestine, and her right ovary and fallopian tube. The cyst that had originally been drained had grown so large that the ovary and tube had to come out. But I was able to keep her uterus and other ovary and tube intact, at least giving her the chance of having children one day.

"I feel like all the people I went to before Dr. Seckin should have been able to give me insight into what was wrong, but they couldn't. The only thing they could say to me was 'hysterectomy,'" Monique said. "In between all those doctor visits, I was in a ton of pain, and the cyst kept growing larger. When I told Dr. Seckin that I was forty years old, he said, 'And they wanted to do a hysterectomy? You're too young!' It was nice to hear a doctor say that. I was touched. He validated what I had always felt: a hysterectomy is not the answer."

Julie felt a colossal amount of pain beginning with her first cycle at age fourteen. But unlike most women with endometriosis, she was diagnosed with it just a year later. "I went to a gynecologist for the first time when I was fifteen, and she did an exam and found a grapefruit-sized cyst on my ovary," Julie said. "She thought I might have endometriosis, but she wasn't sure." The cyst was surgically removed. "When the pain got more intense soon after the surgery, she sent me to a specialist." The specialist initially doubted that Julie had the disease. "She thought I was too young to have it and thought I was being dramatic. She said she would do exploratory surgery, but she was confident she wouldn't find anything. After a five-hour surgery, I woke up and she told me I had it everywhere. I was fifteen years old and was already in stage IV." The specialist burned the disease using laser surgery. Julie's pain remained.

Julie continued to have one laser surgery after another, forcing her to miss large chunks of high school, including three to five months in each of her junior and senior years. She had to rely on a home tutor to help her graduate. One of her surgeries was performed by an endometriosis specialist located nearly nine hundred miles away, whom she was referred to by a family friend. When that surgery didn't work, he recommended a hysterectomy. She was just eighteen years old. The thought of losing her uterus at such a young age was not ideal, but if it would relieve her pain, she felt she would be okay with it.

"I said to him, 'If there is any chance that you can save my uterus, please do,' But when I woke up from surgery, he told me he'd had to remove it. He said there would have been no way I could carry kids anyway because my uterus was in such bad shape," Julie said.

She said she felt some relief for several months after the hysterectomy, and actually felt better than she had since her cycle started. "But six months after the surgery, I started to feel the pain again," Julie said. "It wasn't as bad as before, but it was back. I ended up having three more laser surgeries while I was in college."

After graduating from college, Julie started law school. The pain became unbearable during her first year. "I took a heating pad to my classes and it made a permanent burn mark on my skin because I used it so much. Then I started missing classes, and I finally had to take a medical leave of absence."

She went back to the same doctor who did the hysterectomy, only to have him tell her that he didn't think it was possible she had endometriosis anymore. "I knew that wasn't true," Julie said. "The pain was worse than anything I'd had in high school. They gave me tests, said they were negative, gave me the runaround. I didn't know what to do. I was losing hope."

She found yet another endometriosis specialist, who told her he didn't think the three previous surgeries she'd had were necessary. What was his solution? "Physical therapy," Julie said. "He thought all I needed was a physical therapist. It didn't help, and I only got worse. I was at a loss. I had no idea what to do. I was pretty much physically immobilized."

Her mother's boyfriend, saddened to see her suffering so much, did some research on the Internet and found me. Julie had been to so many doctors in such a short span, none who made her permanently better and some who made her worse, that she wasn't sure what to think of me when she first came in. But I believed she was in as much pain as she claimed, and that she needed serious, immediate help. This alone made her trust me.

"I knew I was in the right place," Julie said. "Dr. Seckin couldn't believe they did a hysterectomy on me when I was only eighteen. He said there was no way he would have done that. He knew what was wrong inside me, and more importantly he knew the right way to treat it. He put me on a treatment plan and clearly explained it, which nobody had ever done. And he had me meet with the other doctors who were going to be part of his team for the surgery. I felt like all the doctors I had gone to previously were quick to do surgery because they made money every time they opened me up. Dr. Seckin was my twelfth surgery. Had the surgery he did been my first, it might have been my only one."

Julie said she has finally come to terms with the fact that she had a hysterectomy at such a young age. "Part of me is still angry about it, but there is nothing I can do. Now that I'm older and know what I know about the disease, I know how crazy it was for that doctor to do that to me. I just want to prevent it from happening to someone else."

She has also come to terms with the fact that it took twelve surgeries for her to get better. "You question your sanity because doctors are questioning your sanity," she said. "I realize this isn't cancer; it doesn't take lives the way cancer does. But, like cancer, it's invasive, it keeps spreading, it causes a lot of pain, and it affects your life and the lives around you in a very deep and personal way. People need to realize that."

A significant number of my patients—probably one in every fifteen or twenty—have already had a hysterectomy by the time they come to me because it's what their doctors recommended, and in most cases it probably wasn't necessary. If your doctor says you need a hysterectomy, don't panic, but trust your instincts and be prepared to defend your uterus. Ask your doctor a lot of questions, and get more opinions, especially if you may want to try to have children one day, because once your uterus is gone, there is no putting it back. Even if you don't want to have children, understand that removing your uterus will not stop the endometriosis or the pain if the disease has spread to other areas. Know definitively what the problem is first, along with all the possible solutions. Then determine your best course of action.

NOTE: See image 12 in the photo section starting on page 93.

17

Appendicitis

THE APPENDIX IS AN ORGAN located on the right side of the abdominal area that, as far as we know, serves no purpose. Appendicitis is an inflammation of the appendix and usually requires a relatively short visit to the emergency room to have it surgically removed. The surgery is so common that it's generally done on an outpatient basis, assuming the organ hasn't ruptured. If it's ruptured, it can cause serious issues in the abdominal cavity that need to be addressed immediately before irreparable damage is done.

Endometriosis is often misdiagnosed by doctors as appendicitis for the same reasons it's often misdiagnosed as IBS. When you consider some of the symptoms of appendicitis—pain in the abdomen area, cramps, gassiness, diarrhea, painful urination, nausea—it's understandable why the misdiagnosis might be made. But many endometriosis patients are brought to the emergency room, where enough care and attention isn't given in order to catch the endometriosis. Doctors who perform an appendectomy because they think appendicitis is the cause of the pain need to have the knowledge to be able to diagnose endometriosis during the surgery. Many doctors who perform appendectomies, usually general surgeons, don't know what endometriosis is, so they wouldn't diagnose it if they were staring right at it (which they often are). It is, in my opinion, an issue of responsibility. When doctors remove an organ, they should recognize a disease that's right in front of them. The unfortunate reality is that often, once the appendix is removed and goes to pathology, the report openly admits that there was no appendicitis. And if appendicitis *is* found in the pathology, the general surgeon will assume nothing else is wrong, and the endometriosis will remain in the areas around the appendix, untreated and not removed.

If endometriosis is not something a doctor can properly treat, he or she should know specialists who can—specifically, physicians who perform deep-excision surgery—and should refer the patient to them. Doctors who do appendectomies and recognize endometriosis often dismiss it as a "woman's disease" and send the patient to her gynecologist (who may not even know what endometriosis is, which is another problem). Endometriosis is not simply a "woman's disease." It's a multi-organ disease affecting women that needs to be identified and treated with a sense of urgency.

In Stephanie's story, you read an example of a lack of urgency on the part of several doctors. One doctor saw a tumor on her appendix, so he removed the appendix. During the surgery, he noticed that she had endometriosis on multiple organs, but rather than refer her to an endometriosis specialist, he sent her back to her gynecologist. The gynecologist didn't have much knowledge of the disease and put her on medication to send her into menopause. That failed to solve the problem. Stephanie went to another OB/GYN, who performed a hysterectomy but left endometriosis tissue on the other organs. Stephanie lost a lot of time, as well as her reproductive organs, to a condition that could have been addressed much sooner by her doctors if they had known more about endometriosis.

If you are diagnosed with appendicitis, it may be just that. It's a common disease. But if you have some of the other symptoms of endometriosis, tell your doctor. If you undergo an appendectomy, make sure your surgeon knows what endometriosis is and request that he or she checks for it during the procedure. If you still experience pain after your appendix has been removed, especially if it continues happening monthly with your cycle, you will know that the chance you have endometriosis has significantly increased. You need to find a doctor who understands the urgency of the situation. Losing your appendix won't hurt you. Losing time to treat the actual problem could.

18

Ovarian Cysts

OVARIAN CYSTS ARE PART OF the ovulation process and occur each month. The cysts, found on the inside of the ovaries, are filled with fluid. Often, the fluid is clear and the cysts are harmless; they usually disappear on their own with no medication. Other times, they can be chocolate cysts—filled with fragments of endometrial tissue, thickened blood, and inflammatory enzymes—which can cause agonizing pain.

If a doctor tells a woman she has a simple ovarian cyst and has nothing to worry about when that cyst is actually an ovarian endometrioma, he or she has just given her an enormous misdiagnosis with potentially devastating repercussions. A chocolate cyst is the root cause of the most advanced endometriosis cases. These cysts rupture and leak during the time of menses and thick, chocolate-like fluid sticks to the intestines and pelvic sidewalls. The fluid later infiltrates these same organs. It is common to see patients with ruptured ovarian cysts in emergency rooms. You read earlier about Michele's doctor telling her that she had a small ovarian cyst and that birth control pills should shrink it (because the pills would reduce the amount of estrogen produced in her body). Six weeks later, after it ruptured, she underwent emergency surgery.

Basira, a patient in her late twenties, had many symptoms of endometriosis, including constipation, painful intercourse, and pain in her legs, lower back, and ovaries. As a nurse, she was familiar with endometriosis and believed that it could be the cause of her symptoms. Her OB/GYN did a sonogram, which revealed a chocolate cyst. The doctor got the diagnosis correct but did not understand the potential severity of it, and he suggested that Basira go on birth control to try to shrink the cyst. Basira did research on chocolate cysts and realized that birth control was not the answer. "I knew that there was absolutely no reason why I should have a blood-filled cyst on my ovary," Basira said. "I knew it was more serious than the doctor thought."

If your doctor tells you that you have a cyst but there's nothing to worry about, start asking questions. The first one should be, "Is it a chocolate cyst?" If the answer is yes, then you absolutely do have something to worry about. It needs to be removed through excision surgery before it ruptures and causes more damage. If the doctor answers, "I don't know," or "I don't think it is," then find a doctor who does know. You can't play roulette with this situation. If it's not a chocolate cyst and you elect to try to treat it through birth control pills or some other method, be sure to have your doctor monitor it, and treat any future cysts with the same diligence with which you treated the first one. Just because the first one wasn't an ovarian endometrioma doesn't mean the next one won't be.

View and download the following pictures in color at
http://www.drseckin.com/the-doctor-will-see-you-now

Surgical view of pelvis

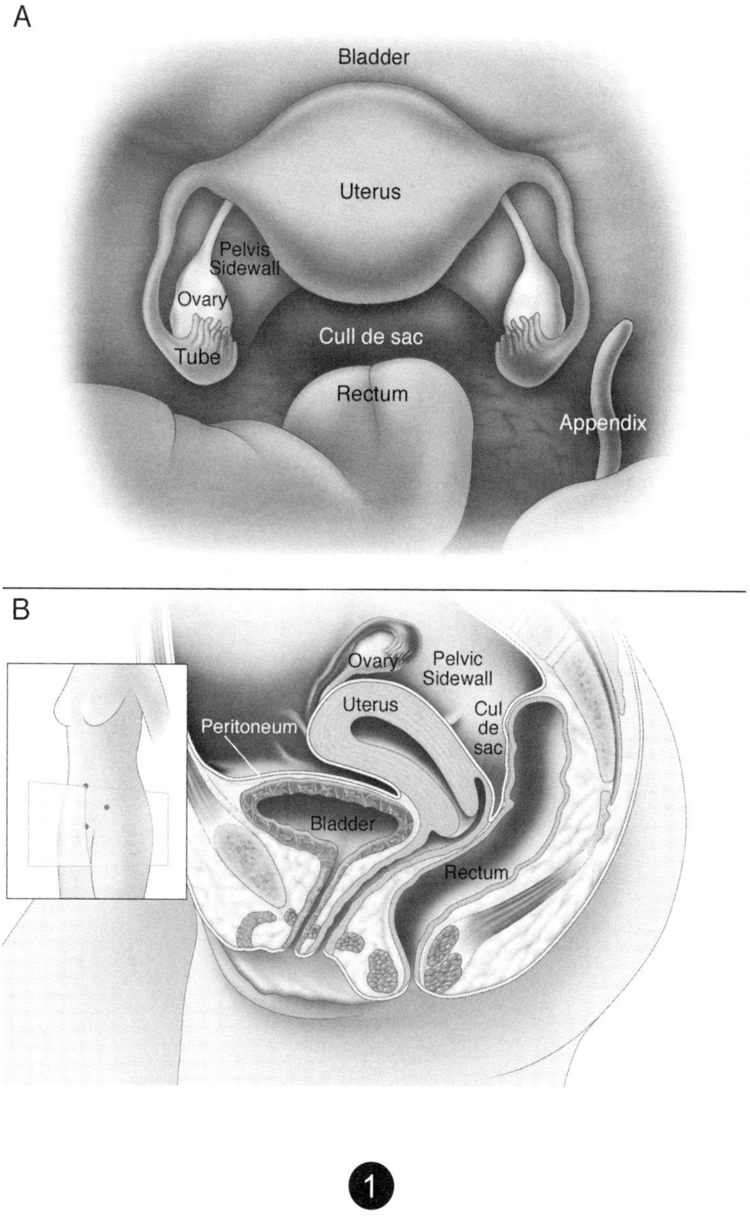

A

Bladder

Uterus

Pelvis Sidewall

Ovary

Tube

Cull de sac

Rectum

Appendix

B

Ovary

Pelvic Sidewall

Uterus

Peritoneum

Cul de sac

Bladder

Rectum

1

TAMER SECKIN, MD

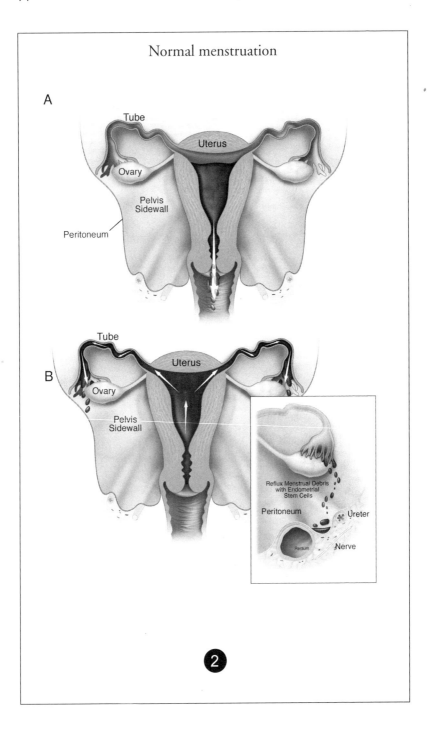

Retrograde menstruation

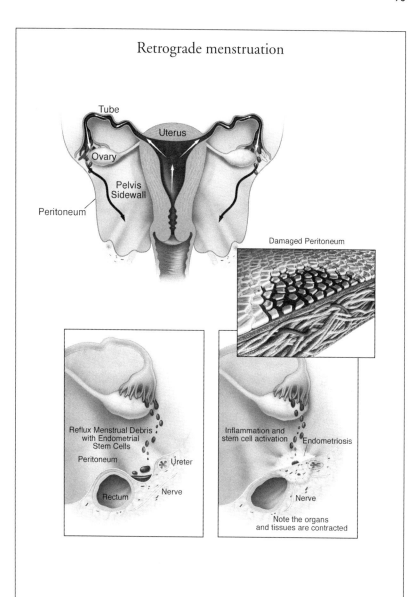

Damaged Peritoneum

Tube
Uterus
Ovary
Pelvis Sidewall
Peritoneum

Reflux Menstrual Debris with Endometrial Stem Cells
Peritoneum
Rectum
Ureter
Nerve

Inflammation and stem cell activation
Endometriosis
Nerve
Note the organs and tissues are contracted

3

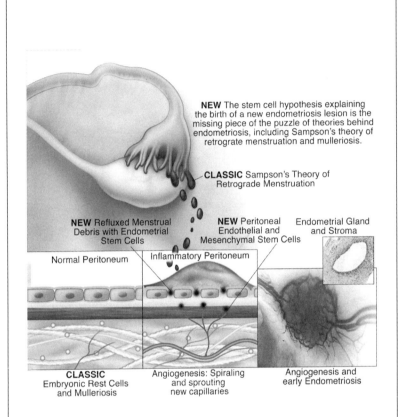

NEW The stem cell hypothesis explaining the birth of a new endometriosis lesion is the missing piece of the puzzle of theories behind endometriosis, including Sampson's theory of retrograte menstruation and mulleriosis.

CLASSIC Sampson's Theory of Retrograde Menstruation

NEW Refluxed Menstrual Debris with Endometrial Stem Cells

NEW Peritoneal Endothelial and Mesenchymal Stem Cells

Endometrial Gland and Stroma

Normal Peritoneum

Inflammatory Peritoneum

CLASSIC Embryonic Rest Cells and Mulleriosis

Angiogenesis: Spiraling and sprouting new capillaries

Angiogenesis and early Endometriosis

4

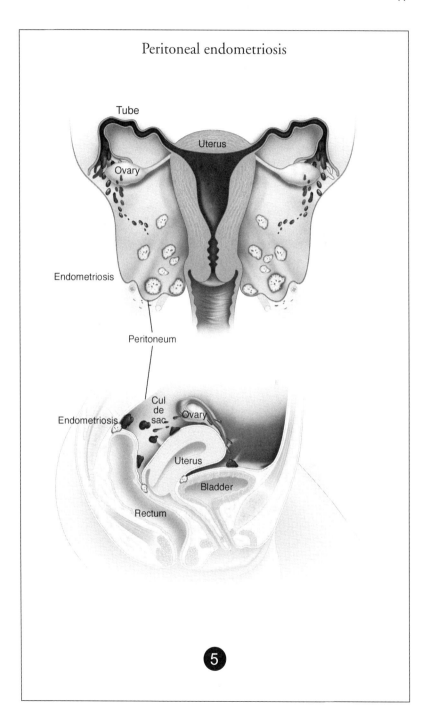

Peritoneal endometriosis

5

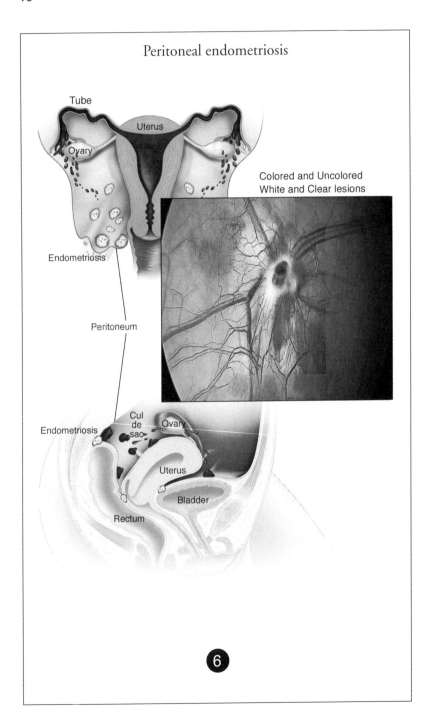

Peritoneal endometriosis

Tube

Uterus

Ovary

Endometriosis

Colored and Uncolored
White and Clear lesions

Peritoneum

Endometriosis

Cul
de
sac

Ovary

Uterus

Bladder

Rectum

6

Peritoneal endometriosis

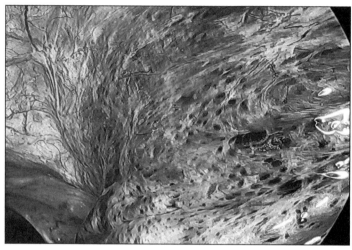

White and clear uncolored
lesions are best recognized
by Aqua Blue Contrast
ABC technique(TM)

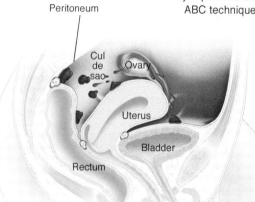

7

Peritoneal endometriosis

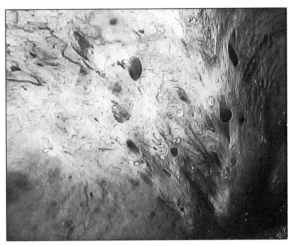

White and clear uncolored
lesions are best recognized
by Dr. Seckin's Aqua Blue Contrast
ABC technique(TM)

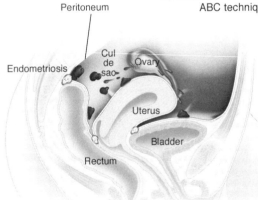

8

Endometrioma

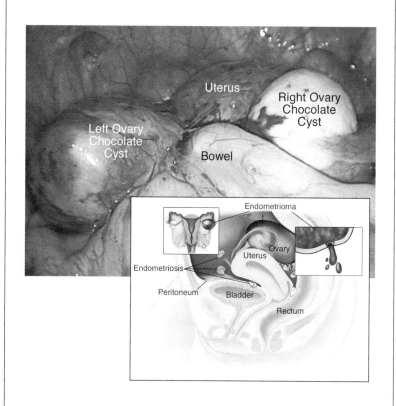

9

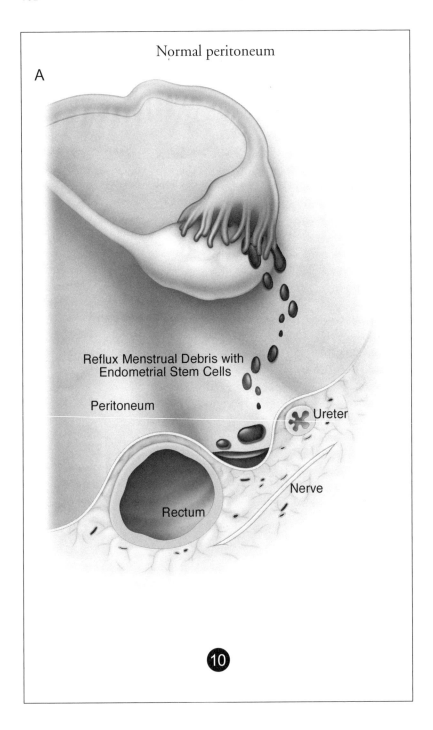

Normal peritoneum

A

Reflux Menstrual Debris with
Endometrial Stem Cells

Peritoneum

Ureter

Nerve

Rectum

10

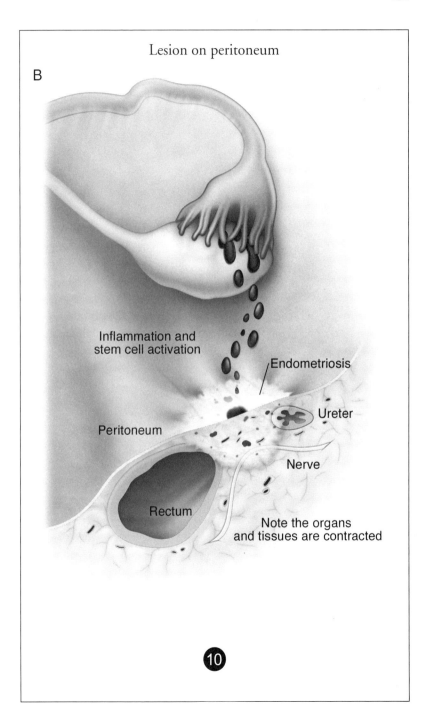

Lesion on peritoneum

B

Inflammation and
stem cell activation

Endometriosis

Ureter

Peritoneum

Nerve

Rectum

Note the organs
and tissues are contracted

10

Deep Infiltrating Endometriosis:
Constipation, painful bowel movements, and diarrhea

A

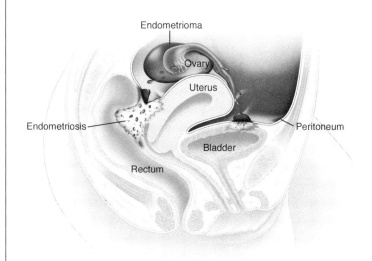

B

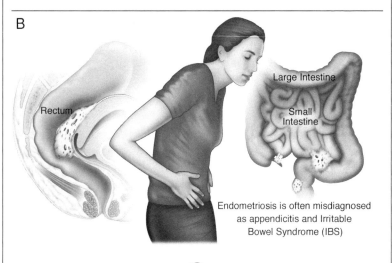

Endometriosis is often misdiagnosed
as appendicitis and Irritable
Bowel Syndrome (IBS)

11

Common conditions causing heavy and painful periods:
Adenomyosis-endometriosis of the uterus,
endometrial polyps, and uterine fibroids

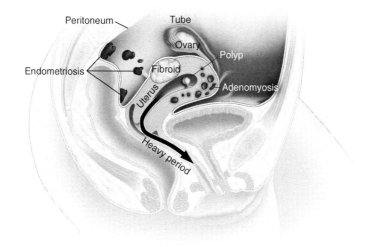

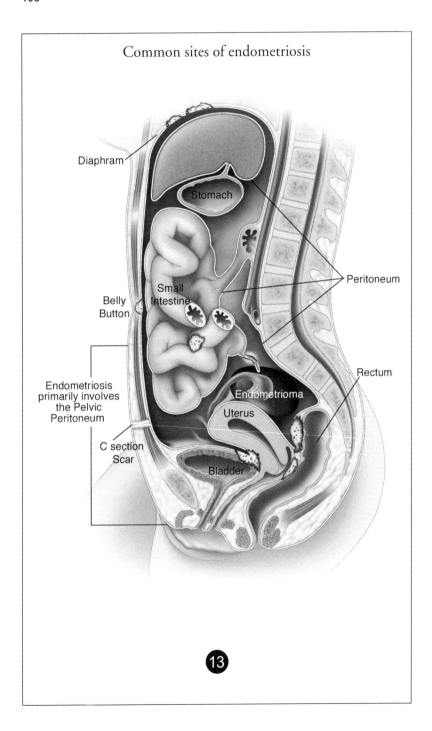

Common sites of endometriosis

Diaphram

Stomach

Peritoneum

Belly
Button

Small
Intestine

Endometriosis
primarily involves
the Pelvic
Peritoneum

Rectum

Endometrioma

Uterus

C section
Scar

Bladder

13

Electric fulguration or coagulation of endometriosis lesion:
Incomplete procedure. Endometriosis left behind.

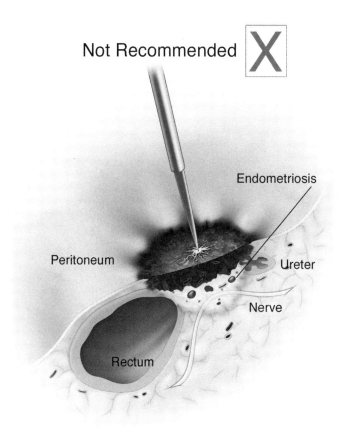

14

Laser ablation of lesion:
Incomplete procedure. Endometriosis left behind.

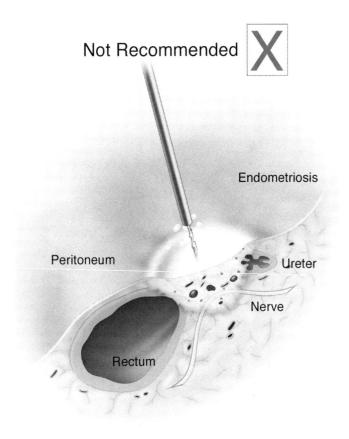

Not Recommended X

Endometriosis

Peritoneum

Ureter

Nerve

Rectum

15

Excision of lesion:
Complete procedure. No Endometriosis left behind.

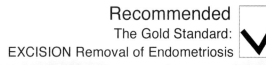

Recommended
The Gold Standard:
EXCISION Removal of Endometriosis

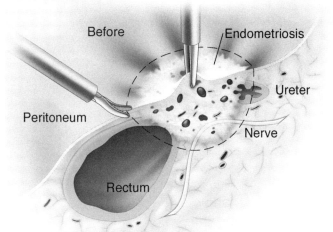

Before

Endometriosis

Ureter

Peritoneum

Nerve

Rectum

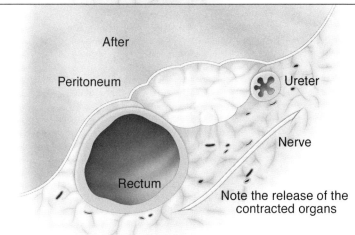

After

Peritoneum

Ureter

Nerve

Rectum

Note the release of the
contracted organs

16

Painful sex

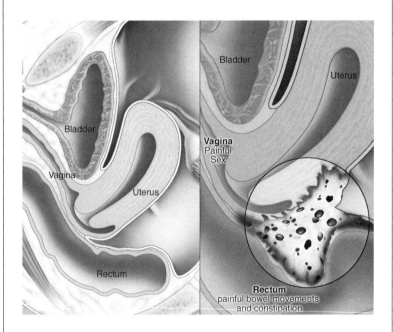

17

Effects

19

Those Who Suffer with Them

YOU MET TOM, LAUREN'S HUSBAND, at the beginning of this book, and you learned how difficult it was for him to watch his wife suffer for so many years. As I've stated, no man, or woman without endometriosis, will ever know the physical trials a woman goes through with endometriosis, but when it's his or her partner or mother or daughter, he or she suffers emotionally with her because of the deep love for her.

Drew knows that feeling all too well. His wife, Carissa, had endometriosis for about twenty-five years before finding me in 2015. During those years she suffered severe symptoms of the disease, was misdiagnosed, and, after she was finally diagnosed by another doctor, went through dreaded laser surgery. In those respects it was a classic case of endometriosis. Also typical was that she had a partner suffering behind the scenes with her. Drew and Carissa have been married for ten years. They have been together for about twelve years. They have two young children. (Fortunately, and surprisingly, infertility was not one of the symptoms that struck Carissa.) Drew said that after my surgery on his wife, "We have our lives back." But getting their lives back was something he thought might never happen.

"You look at a woman like my wife who is so independent, so motivated, a go-getter who takes care of me and the kids and her job, who never complains and never takes a sick day. When she is going through something like this and you don't know what it is or where to turn, it's so tough," Drew said. "I always try my best to make sure everything is good for her, to take any burdens off her. And when I can't, it drives me insane because there is nothing I can do. That's the effect this disease had on me."

Drew said Carissa's endometriosis took away everything that was good in their lives. "It took away our emotional life and our sexual life. It took a mother away from her kids because Mommy couldn't get on the ground to play with them or run after them for a quick hug or give them a bath. I was losing not only my wife, but my best friend. There is nothing worse than seeing the one you love just get through life. You don't think it's going to get any better because you can't see a light at the end of the tunnel."

Drew said he knew that something wasn't physically right with Carissa. Growing up with his mother and sister, he never remembered either of them going through anything close to what Carissa dealt with. "She would have pain for ten days. I told her that wasn't normal, but she said that's just how it is, so I thought, 'Okay, I'm out of it. She knows what she is talking about.' " Carissa's information came from the usual sources: women close to her who thought her pain was nothing more than the regular result of periods and doctors who didn't consider endometriosis as a possibility or even know what it was.

During her two pregnancies, Carissa got a bit of a break from the effects of endometriosis since she wasn't menstruating. But after the second child was born, the pain attacked again with a vengeance. "She didn't want to go out and do anything," Drew said. "I felt so bad for her. She couldn't go to the pool in the summer. We'd have to strategically plan our vacation to the shore based on her cycle. Our life was always based on how she would feel."

I have seen this disease tear relationships apart. But as much as Drew and Carissa's marriage suffered emotionally, they navigated their way through it. "I just resigned myself to the fact that this was the way life was going to be. It was just the hand we were dealt," Drew said. "It was definitely an intense ride."

That changed once Carissa received the proper diagnosis, learned what endometriosis was, and underwent deep-excision surgery. Now she is pain free, and they've rebuilt their lives. Drew said there needs to be across-the-board education about endometriosis—for young girls, women, men, doctors, and nurses—so that nobody has to suffer through what he and Carissa endured. "There needs to be some kind of intervention or screening or education where everybody knows what 'normal' looks like. A lot of women have endometriosis and don't know it. I'm six-foot-five, but I felt about two feet tall when my wife was going through this and I had no idea what to do for her. When it comes to family, you decide that you will just find a way to make things better, but with a health issue like this, if you don't know what it is, you can't do anything about it."

Drew's sentiments echo those of Tom, Lauren's husband, who said the disease made him feel helpless as a partner. He also said that as hard as it can be, you have to realize that your partner needs you more than ever during that difficult time. "To anyone whose wife or girlfriend is going through this, I would say you need to be very understanding, and you need to always be there for her," Tom said. "This disease does not discriminate, and it does not make her less of a woman. You may not be able to have children, but don't pin that on her. Just try to understand what she is going through and be patient. Also know that after surgery, it can take a while for her to mend. Just encourage her to relax and to take it one day at a time."

20

Living Just to Work

BUSINESSES LOSE BILLIONS OF DOLLARS each year to the devastating effects of endometriosis on employees. That said, many women with endometriosis remain incredibly hardworking and refuse to let their pain keep them from completing their responsibilities. I've observed that my patients are honest, reliable women who do not want to miss work, and don't miss work, especially when the alternative is to call in sick with a condition they cannot or do not want to explain. To repeat what Padma said about the challenges of continuing to work with endometriosis, "I just did not want to tell people why, because it is really embarrassing to talk about your period, especially when you are a young girl. It is really not fun. Not to your boyfriend, not to the editor who has hired you for the lingerie job, not to anybody really." Furthermore, endometriosis patients typically don't look sick. If women with endometriosis claim to be sick, they are doubted. If they try to hide their disease and work through it, they are miserable. They can't win either way.

Carissa, whose husband, Drew, you met in the last chapter, is a pediatric occupational therapist. To this day, she has no idea how she survived in the workplace before she underwent surgery:

> I worked with children with special needs six days a week back then. They ranged in age from birth to thirteen years old and had autism or various

physical disabilities. It wasn't like a desk job where you could take a break for a brief period without anyone knowing what you were going through. I was always on my feet working hands-on with the kids and their parents. I had a new appointment every half hour and had to always be on top of my game. If I had to cancel on those kids, they wouldn't understand. And if I didn't work, I didn't get paid. I really have no idea how I did it. I felt like I was going insane. If I said anything about how I felt, people thought I was making it up because I looked fine. They had no idea what was going on inside of me. It was so challenging to have to deal with that. I didn't feel like I could talk about it with anybody except my husband. He was the only one who understood me.

Carissa took a lot of ibuprofen and used heating pads every chance she could. She wore black pants each day to help cover up any blood from her period. She was also careful about how she scheduled her clients. "I never scheduled babies for back-to-back appointments because I knew I wouldn't be able to physically handle it," she said. "If I was working with a baby, I knew there were certain positions I couldn't get into or the pain would be too much. If I hadn't been working so closely with children, I definitely would have taken those days off, but those kids were counting on me every day. I didn't know what else to do. I just accepted that my life was always going to be that way. I wasn't living; I was just getting through it."

Annie Rose is another patient who rarely took a sick day. Over a ten-year period working for the state of New Jersey, she could always be counted on to be there. All her appointments with various doctors were scheduled on her own time. If she felt awful, then she felt awful at work, and she still found a way to effectively do her job. One time her pain was so severe that she had to be taken to the hospital straight from work. A couple of days later she was back at her job—still in pain and with no diagnosis. But she knew no other way. "I would come home at 7:30 each night, pass out on the couch, and do it again the next day. I don't know how I did it. I was living just to work."

Immediately prior to her surgery with me, Annie Rose's pain was so overwhelming that she had to start using her sick time. By the time she entered her recovery period after surgery, her sick days were gone and she had to go on disability. "I watched a whole ten years of accrued sick time go away with endometriosis," she said. "You see some people abuse their sick time to spend the day at the beach. I was too dedicated to do that. And I eventually needed every sick day I had because of this disease."

Elissa, the single mother of three who had a four-hour round-trip commute each day, worked as an administrative assistant at a law firm, a job that required a lot of interaction with people. But she tried to never let her pain show, which created additional issues for her. "People would look at me and say, 'You don't look sick. You look healthy. I don't understand why you feel the way you say you do.' They almost make you feel like it's in your head," she said. "I was always in pain, always tired. I missed a lot of work because of my doctor appointments, and it was difficult to take that time off. My bosses weren't happy about it. They just didn't understand how bad this was."

Beth, who shared her story about painful sex, was a brand strategist for a major television network and later for one of the world's largest social-media companies. She did everything possible to prevent the endometriosis symptoms from taking over her work. "I was always in a lot of pain," she said. "The only way I could get through each work day was with pain medication and by trying to focus on my work even more." When she reached a point at which she knew the disease was about to take over her job, she elected to undergo surgery with me. In the end, she became healthy, but there were costs along the way. "I never let it affect my work, but when I came home at night, I was done," she said. "I had to cancel any plans I had with friends."

You will read more in the next chapter about the rifts in friendships this disease caused for Beth and others. None of the women in this chapter, or any of the thousands of other patients of mine whose work has been affected by endometriosis, ever adopted a "woe is me" attitude, even though they had every right to feel that way. The stories about how this disease impacted their work or social lives or family lives are ones they don't normally tell others. They shared them for this book as a favor to me, and ultimately as a favor to you, because they don't want you to experience what they experienced. They don't want you to have to deal with bosses who don't understand or a company that doesn't care. They don't want you to be questioned by your managers or coworkers about how sick you really are just because you don't look sick. They don't want your dream career to vanish because of this disease. Lauren told you about losing a shot at her dream job with the US Postal Inspection Service because of endometriosis. Listen to her and to the rest of these women.

21

You Learn Who Your True Friends Are

ENDOMETRIOSIS CAN BE RUTHLESS TOWARD a woman's social life. Besides causing problems in her romantic relationships, it can reveal who her true friends are. Some diseases, such as cancer, bring out the best in friends, prompting them to show great levels of support to a friend or loved one who's been diagnosed. By contrast, women living with the symptoms of endometriosis—whether or not they've been diagnosed yet—often don't receive the same kind of love and concern. This is largely due to the lack of awareness surrounding the disease. For many endometriosis sufferers, some social connections have been irreparably broken.

For Annie Rose, it started when she was a teenager, got worse as the years went on, and occasionally remains a problem today. "I've been misunderstood for more than half my life," she said. "It began when I was thirteen. I would tell my friends that I was bleeding heavily or that the pain was just too much. They'd say, 'My God, your periods are that bad?' I'd say, 'Yeah, they're that bad.' They'd say, 'Oh whatever. It's just your period.' And they'd tell me that every woman gets it and I just needed to get over it."

When Annie Rose was in her late twenties and still didn't have a correct diagnosis, the attitudes of her friends hadn't changed. If anything, they became colder. "They'd say, 'Oh, she's making excuses again not to go out. She's got depression.' Having this disease can certainly lead to depression, but that's not what I had. I didn't know what it was, but I knew it was a physical disease inside me. The pain and inflammation wore me out. But they said, 'Hey, we keep asking you out, but if you keep turning us down, we're not going to ask anymore.' "

Annie Rose was finally diagnosed with endometriosis in her early thirties. "And believe it or not, some of my friends became even more ignorant after the diagnosis," she said. "They'd say, 'Okay, if you have it, then just get a hysterectomy.' They thought that would cure me, but there is no cure. And a hysterectomy wasn't going to make me better. They just didn't understand."

She said some of her friends put the blame for the disease on her shoulders by telling her that she had it because she hadn't had any children. "I know if it was one of my friends suffering from this, I would have been more supportive, and I certainly would have never said anything like that," Annie Rose said. "This disease really destroyed a lot of my friendships. You learn with this disease who your true friends are."

For many years, Beth pushed through her pain when she had plans with friends or family. "My dad's a Marine. We don't complain about this kind of stuff. We just deal with it," Beth said. But when she reached her late twenties, after suffering with the disease for more than fifteen years, she often had to cancel on loved ones. "I remember one Easter we were supposed to visit my husband's family, but I just couldn't," she said. "My husband understood, but I still felt guilty about it."

"When I turned twenty-eight I started being honest with people and telling them why I couldn't do things," Beth continued. "Before that, I just pushed through it, but I couldn't suck it up anymore. Most people understood, but I know I also lost a lot of friends because of it. My attitude is that they were not real friends if they couldn't understand how bad it was for me. I really focused on investing in the relationships I cared about, with the people who cared about me, and because of that I have such close friendships today. You definitely lose friends because of this disease, but you also have the opportunity to develop stronger bonds with people."

Jessica, whom you met in the chapter on neuropathy, also understands the value of those strong bonds. "When you get a flare-up from the endometriosis, you can't go out, you can't do anything," she said. "When you're younger, you think that's the end of the world, but I was fortunate that I always had a good group of friends who understood what I was dealing with. If I had to cancel, they understood. No matter what the situation was, I had their backs, and they had mine."

I think these three amazing women offer the perfect advice regarding friendships: as you battle this disease and learn who your true friends are, focus on making those friendships stronger and let the other ones go. True friends are not going to doubt that you are telling them the truth. And if you know someone who has this disease or who might have it, understand that she needs you now more than ever. Do not question her or doubt her. Help her. Listen to her. As Jessica said, make sure she knows that you have her back. Most important, believe her.

22

A Miscarriage

YOU'VE MET LAURA, THE PATIENT who experienced so much physical pain in high school that I referred to her heating pads and painkillers as her teddy bears. As is usually the case with my patients, Laura also endured severe emotional trauma from endometriosis, especially when she tried to have a baby. Fertility issues are some of the most heartbreaking effects of this disease. Laura felt it was critical to share her story with you to help you understand the importance of early detection and of finding a doctor who will treat the disease the way it should be treated.

Laura started getting endometriosis symptoms when she was thirteen, and they worsened as the years progressed. She was about nineteen when her doctor performed surgery to remove a cyst from one of her ovaries. As it turned out, the doctor removed an entire ovary and most of the other one because of all the endometriosis she found. Laura underwent several more surgeries over the next ten years, all of them laser, and none of which had any long-term positive effects.

Laura got married in 2009, and she and her husband wanted to have a child. They tried for several months to get pregnant, but couldn't. When Laura went to a reproductive endocrinologist, he told her that her best option was in vitro fertilization.

"I left his office crying," Laura said. "I didn't go in there expecting to hear that. Honestly, I didn't know what to expect. I was only twenty-nine.

I knew endometriosis could cause infertility, but it wasn't until that visit that the reality hit me." Laura initially decided against IVF, but after about six more months of trying unsuccessfully to get pregnant, she sought a second opinion from another endocrinologist.

"He said my ovary wasn't great, but he could do in vitro with hormones," Laura said. "We decided to try it." She said she yielded only three eggs the first time; the doctor was expecting at least ten, and maybe as many as twenty or twenty-five. Two of those three did not fertilize properly, so only one fertilized egg could be inserted into her uterus. It didn't work. They tried again. This time there were four eggs. Two were placed in her uterus, and the placement was successful. She became pregnant. But, devastatingly, she had a miscarriage, and Laura almost lost her own life. "I was about nine weeks pregnant. It was a Saturday, and my husband was working. I felt sick. I thought that just came with being pregnant. But then I started bleeding, and I got a stabbing, burning feeling in my right thigh. I called the doctor and told him something wasn't right. By the time I got to his office, I couldn't stand. I was nauseous. They ended up having to do emergency surgery on me. They found cysts hemorrhaging all around my ovary, and my pregnancy was ectopic."

In a normal pregnancy, an egg is released by the ovary into the fallopian tube. Once fertilized, the egg moves into the uterus, where it continues to grow. In an ectopic pregnancy, the egg implants somewhere outside of the uterus. In Laura's case, because of the endometriosis, the egg was pushed back into the fallopian tube, where it could have caused the tube to burst.

"The surgery lasted three hours, and I was told I came close to not surviving it," Laura said. "It ended my pregnancy, and nearly ended my life."

Laura saw a therapist to help her through the psychological distress. The therapist suggested she find an endometriosis specialist, which led Laura to me. I performed a six-hour surgery that resulted in her being pain free for the first time in more than sixteen years. But her chances of having a baby were almost none. "I'm 95 percent sure I couldn't have a child if we tried because I only have part of my right ovary, and it doesn't function very well in terms of producing healthy eggs," Laura said. "Had I gone to Dr. Seckin first, things might have been different with regard to getting pregnant, but I don't know. I never thought of going to someone like him to begin with, so I don't dwell on it."

Laura has the perfect attitude about the cards she was dealt. What's happened has happened, and there was nothing she could have done differently. She didn't know for several years that she had the symptoms of endometriosis, and she didn't know how it should be treated. But when patients have recurrent miscarriages, we must consider endometriosis as a potential cause. That's why our efforts to create awareness about the disease are so important. Know the symptoms. Know how a doctor should treat those symptoms. Would I have removed one of Laura's ovaries and most of the other one, as the first surgeon did? I can't say for sure, but it's highly likely that, with proper surgical techniques, her ovaries could have been preserved. As I've said previously, if you have any doubts about how your doctor is handling your case, trust your instincts. Ask a lot of questions until you have the answers you need. And know that you are not alone.

Alternatives

23

Alternatives, Not Substitutes

YOU NOW HAVE A SOLID understanding of what endometriosis is, its symptoms, the common misdiagnoses that could delay proper treatment, and the devastating effects it can have on every aspect of a woman's life if not treated in a timely manner. So now what? Now is when you need to see an endometriosis specialist who is an expert in deep-excision surgery and who can restore you to good health. That's the topic of the section that follows, "The Care You Deserve." But before that, in this section, I want to address some possible alternatives to deep-excision surgery. Please note that these are alternatives, not substitutes. Let me explain.

There are alternatives for everything. For the car you have, the house you live in, the place you work, the school you attend, the food you eat, your daily exercise routine, the social media you use, the television shows you watch, the candidates you vote for. You get the picture. But when top-notch quality matters, you can't always substitute one thing for another. For example, you could choose to attend a different school, but if that other school does not have the same level of quality teachers that your current school has, the other school is no substitute. If you are offered a new job, but it cannot match what is important to you in your current job, such as salary or health benefits, the potential new job is an alternative to the one you have but not a substitute.

Likewise, there are alternatives to treating endometriosis with deep-excision surgery, but none of them are substitutes for the correct type of surgery. That goes for the alternatives described in this section as well as the alternatives suggested by doctors or other medical professionals. No alternatives will rid you of long-term pain as effectively as deep-excision surgery will. None of them will prevent the endometriosis from progressing. Some of them may help slow its growth, but they won't stop it or kill the tissue that has already implanted inside your body.

So why even present these alternatives? For several reasons.

Because not every girl with a symptom or two of endometriosis should undergo surgery at age thirteen or fourteen. Alternative methods for controlling the symptoms could give her body time to grow and strengthen before we know for sure that surgery is necessary.

Because not every woman can afford surgery. Some women don't have health insurance. Others do, but it doesn't always cover as much as they need it to cover. It's unfortunate that the health care we receive is often based not on what we need but on what we can afford. That, however, is the reality of the system. If a woman knows she cannot afford surgery now, but thinks she will be able to in a year or two and can safely manage the disease with an alternative therapy in the meantime, then why not try that route?

Because some women are afraid to have surgery and will try any alternative method before considering letting a doctor perform an invasive procedure.

Because some women have recently gone through a pregnancy, or have undergone one or more surgeries for endometriosis or something else, and they want to give their bodies a break.

Because some women have tried alternative therapies that worked for other diseases or conditions they had, or they know people who have successfully done so, and they want to exhaust all other options before considering surgery.

The most important aspect of alternative therapies that you need to be aware of, and that I will reiterate throughout these chapters, is that there is no one-size-fits-all approach with any of them. What works well for one person may not work at all for another. When my patients went to doctors before me and were prescribed some of these alternatives, the results varied. For some, birth control worked well. For others, it did nothing. For some, going into menopause served its purpose. For others, it was a nightmare of side effects that they would never want to experience again. Some got by for years with painkillers. For others, the painkillers may as well have been sugar pills. But, again, no matter what alternative you choose, know that the endometriosis that was inside of you before you started the therapy is still going to be there, is likely still growing, and likely will not stop growing no matter what alternative therapy you try.

Remember what I said early in the book: pain is an instinctive vital sign. It is the brain's perception that something is wrong. If the alternative therapy you try does not help you physically or emotionally, stop using it. Using alternative therapies offers you the time for a personalized approach that may suit only you. Listen to what your body is telling you. And remember that nothing is a substitute for deep-excision surgery that will get rid of the inflammation tissue lodged in your body.

24

Painkillers

PAINKILLERS ARE DRUGS THAT ARE supposed to do just that: kill the pain. It's the option many doctors and patients elect to try first when confronting endometriosis pain. As with pain you experience from any cause—a headache, an earache, a backache—you usually reach for the pill in the medicine cabinet that will give you some temporary relief. But because every person's level of endometriosis pain is different, and because the chemical makeup of people's bodies is different (to a certain extent), the type of painkiller that works (if anything does), the dosage, and the frequency with which it is taken vary from person to person.

A nonsteroidal anti-inflammatory drug such as ibuprofen that is taken based on the recommended dosage and frequency listed on the label may work for one person but have absolutely no effect on another. Sara expressed in an earlier chapter that she ended up on the floor if she didn't have her pain medication. "As a teenager, I took ibuprofen anytime the cramps were bad because that's what my doctors told me to do," she said. "It was just over-the-counter stuff, nothing ever stronger than that, and only during my period. It always helped because the pain was debilitating. It enabled me to at least get up and move around. It didn't make me feel great, but it made me feel better."

Eve, who said the pain from her cramps would "literally knock me off my feet," tried several different pain medications but never found one that consistently worked. "I couldn't just take a couple of aspirin and put this behind me," she said. "I went through a ton of different medications, some of them in high doses, but the pain was too strong for them to have any effect."

One of my youngest patients is Diana, on whom I performed surgery when she was sixteen. Diana was unable to get off her couch during her menstrual period. She had an array of endometriosis symptoms, including killer cramps, nausea, diarrhea, and vomiting. "I missed an entire week of school every month because of my period," Diana said. "The school sent letters to my house about my absences, and my mom would have to explain that I had this problem that nobody could diagnose."

Doctors continually misdiagnosed her—appendicitis, gas, ovarian cysts. Everything, it seemed, except endometriosis. They prescribed painkillers for her to take during her period, but they didn't work. "I actually think the prescribed painkillers made it worse because they would relieve the pain for only two hours before it came back," Diana said. "So the medication would wear off before I was allowed to take more, but I couldn't take something over-the-counter either because the prescription medication was still in my system."

Doctors also had her try taking the prescribed medication the week before she got her period. "That didn't help, either," Diana said. "I would get nauseous and dizzy and tired, and I had to go to school feeling like that. My body just did not react well to those pills. They really messed me up. The only thing I found that consistently helped was taking four Advil every four hours for five straight days accompanied with a heating pad. But that just destroyed my stomach."

A major issue with narcotic pain medication is the risk of dependency and addiction. Addiction to prescription opiates has become an epidemic. Diana did not have that problem, but when the pain is so awful that a person has to take several pills every few hours for several days just to get through it, the risk of addiction greatly increases.

Remember that painkillers are meant to kill the pain. They don't kill endometriosis or do anything to stop it from spreading. In fact, they often cause fatigue and constipation. They are meant to be a temporary fix to get you through your day or a particular situation, such as debilitating menstrual pain. Always listen to your body when you ingest any drug, and pay attention to the dosage and the frequency with which you are taking it.

I recommend that you stay away from prescribed narcotic pain medications because of the potential for addiction and accidental overdoses, and because I believe they kill the function of brain cells even when taken as prescribed, but I also know that doctors are going to continue to prescribe them and patients are going to continue to want them. I have unfortunately seen morphine patches prescribed to a twelve-year-old pubertal girl in an effort to ease her menstrual pain. Please consider the following guidelines if you do take prescribed narcotic pain medications: if the painkiller has no effect on the pain, stop taking it; if your pain has gone away or is manageable, stop taking it; if the side effects are worse to deal with than the pain itself, stop taking it; and if you feel that you need to take a higher dosage than prescribed, don't take it upon yourself to do so—consult your doctor. A person in debilitating pain isn't always thinking clearly. She has one mission, which is to stop the pain, and sometimes at any cost. Let your doctor decide how much is safe to take. He or she may have another type of medication you can try, or he or she may recommend another alternative, such as the ones you will read about in the next few chapters.

25

Acupuncture

THERE IS A COMMON GOAL between all forms of medicine: to cure or improve disease and minimize any aftereffects of the disease. Curing a disease is achieved by helping the body return to its state of harmony, the condition known as homeostasis. One way to help achieve homeostasis is with acupuncture.

At times, acupuncture may appear as being miraculous, but it's not. Acupuncture is a whole system of treatment, unique to itself, that has been helping people heal from all types of diseases for at least three thousand years. Acupuncture, according to *Webster's* dictionary, is the "Chinese practice of inserting fine needles through the skin at specific points, especially to cure disease or relieve pain." Though acupuncture certainly does not rid the body of endometriosis, it is an effective method of treating the symptoms of the disease.

Acupuncture is an energetic medicine that has proven itself through its own scientific methodology. This process originated in China, spread throughout Asia, and eventually throughout the rest of the world. Many different techniques of acupuncture have been developed, but all styles stem from the original Chinese theories. Through trial, error, and the help of some practitioners who were highly attuned to the body's energy pathways, a systematic approach to diagnosis and treatments for patterns of disease evolved. Acupuncture is based on energy flow concepts. These connections are intertwined throughout the body using numerous energetic channels that supply the endpoint organs. When the energy is flowing harmoniously through the channels and organs, homeostasis is present with no symptoms of disease. Along these energetic channels there are specific points that have certain functionality in helping the harmonious flow of energy.

When any symptoms arise, there is disharmony in the system. Depending on the type, location, and quality of the symptoms, these relate accordingly to specific channels and organs. A thorough investigation with specific diagnostic techniques is conducted in order to reveal the disharmony in the patient. Depending on the diagnosis, an acupuncture point prescription is administered to the patient. The insertion of metal needles into these specific points, using a certain technique, helps the body regulate the energetic disharmony. The body's natural mechanism is to be in homeostasis, and acupuncture helps the body remember how to achieve this function. The number of treatments and the effectiveness of the treatments will be determined by the severity and the longevity of the disharmony.

Endometriosis is a complex disease that is associated with chronic pelvic pain, especially when it has been misdiagnosed or when incomplete surgical removal has occurred. Acupuncture can be of significant benefit to these patients. The most prevalent symptoms of endometriosis that acupuncture treats are pain, reduction of mass size and surrounding tissue inflammation, and infertility. Acupuncture can help treat these conditions, as an adjunctive therapy with no side effects. Acupuncture has had success as the sole method used in treating endometriosis and in keeping a patient less symptomatic. However, in current times, a combined approach is always favorable for best outcomes. It is very important to achieve a correct diagnosis using patient history and a physical exam, radiological evaluation, and laparoscopy. Surgical excision of the disease is the optimal treatment.

The most important symptom that acupuncture can help with is controlling the associated pelvic pain syndromes. It can be a very cost-effective way of treating pain without the side effects you may experience with hormone therapy and narcotics.

So how does acupuncture treat pain?

The energetic pathways that are used in acupuncture run close to the nervous system. When there is pain in a healthy homeostatic body, the normal condition is for the brain to recognize the pain and then release enkephalins, endorphins, and other strong pain-relieving substances. The nerve impulse is then relieved of the sensation of pain. In the case of chronic pain, a condition we often see with endometriosis, the brain-to-pain connection is often lost. What happens over time with chronic pain in a certain area is that the nerves start to lose connectivity to the brain. The nociceptors, or sensory nerves, sense there is pain but cannot localize where it is coming from. Over time, that peripheral nerve or pro-prioceptor's ability to communicate with the brain becomes debilitated. Inserting needles helps the nerves improve their signal strength in order to communicate properly with the brain. The brain can then improve connection with the appropriate area of the body. Electro stimulation can also be connected to the acupuncture needles. Using certain electrical frequencies further helps the nervous system out of pain and inflammation. This concept is also prevalent in medicine with neurostimulator devices marketed for epilepsy and chronic back pain. However, keep in mind that increasing electrical current flow through acupuncture needles is not effective for endometriosis patients.

In terms of treating infertility, if a patient does not want or cannot have hormone therapy, she can consider acupuncture as an effective alternative treatment. There are many documented case studies in which acupuncture was successful as the sole treatment for infertility, and the literature is extensive regarding Chinese patterns of disease associated with infertility. Given the enduring history of acupuncture, it may be an alternative treatment worth trying. Like the other alternatives, it won't make the endometriosis disappear or prevent it from spreading, but it may make the pain more tolerable and help improve fertility until you can get the endometriosis treated.

26

Good Nutrition

AS ONE OF MY PATIENTS, Casey, was leaving her initial appointment with me, I gave her some nutritional advice. "I remember Dr. Seckin saying to me, 'Remember, no gluten or dairy, eat organic, and try to stay away from sugar, caffeine, and red meat.' At that moment, my whole world changed," Casey said. "I shouldn't have been too surprised that endometriosis and diet were connected, but I was. It never crossed my mind. Furthermore, after talking to many women in the endometriosis community, they verified that they, too, felt better after staying away from certain foods. Many women, through the process of trial and elimination, had figured out just what Dr. Seckin had told me."

What constitutes "good nutrition" varies from person to person because no two bodies are exactly the same. Like painkillers, what works well for one person may not work well for another. But we do know that, generally speaking, good nutrition is about minimizing toxins and maximizing nutrients. Relieving pain, reducing inflammation, bolstering the immune system, balancing hormones, and lessening stress are achieved by providing the body with nutritional support.

Begin your journey toward good nutrition by developing an awareness of how you feel after you have eaten something. If you eat something and cannot go to sleep afterward, try to determine what you ate that could be keeping you awake. If you eat lunch and you feel bloated afterward, it may not be the best lunch for you. Even if all you have is a salad and a bottle of water, that salad may not be the right food for your body. As you do when dealing with pain, listen to your body. If a part of your body is telling you that it doesn't want a certain food, you would be smart to remove that food from your diet.

Endometriosis patients should consider decreasing or eliminating inflammatory foods, such as white sugar, dairy products, common cooking oils, trans fats, deep-fried foods, processed foods, red meat, alcohol, and wheat. Artificial food additives or any foods that cause an allergic reaction, including gluten-containing foods, can cause problems for some people. So can coffee and tobacco products. Also be careful of nonorganic, nongrass-fed meats because of the added growth hormones they contain.[xiii]

I know—these guidelines eliminate a lot of foods you probably love. I didn't say this would be easy. No lifestyle change is. But when you consider the benefits a change in diet may be able to bring you with regard to endometriosis, I believe it's worth trying.

Some anti-inflammatory foods you can add to your diet include the particularly antioxidant power of cumin and turmeric, both from the ginger family. Other antioxidant foods are berries (especially blueberries), pineapple, papaya, broccoli, cauliflower, sweet potatoes, extra-virgin olive oil, coconut oil, shiitake mushrooms, wild-caught salmon, green tea, pistachios, walnuts, almonds, and chestnuts. Other good foods, especially during your menstrual cycle, include dark-green leafy vegetables, beets, sprouts, legumes, dates, figs, and apricots. Organic meats and eggs can also be very nourishing.[xiv]

"It is really hard eating gluten-free, dairy-free, organic, and staying away from caffeine, alcohol, and most sugar," Casey said. "There are times I do really well with what I eat. There are other times when I do not do as well and pay the price for eating as I wish. Can eating right cure my endometriosis? No, but I do feel that when I eat right, my quality of life improves dramatically."

Ultimately, there is no conclusive magical endometriosis diet that works for everyone, but the measures you take to reduce inflammations can alleviate symptoms. As always, listen to your body. Pay attention to how you feel after eating a certain food or drinking a certain drink. Like Casey said, what you eat or don't eat is not going to cure endometriosis, but good nutrition could have a positive effect on the pain you feel by reducing inflammation and balancing your hormones.

27

Birth Control Pills

WHEN THE NAME IMPLIES THAT the purpose of the pill is to control birth, it's understandable that there would be a lack of education on what else the pill can do for a woman and her health.

In a nutshell, birth control pills, most of which contain the hormones estrogen and progestin, prevent a woman's ovaries from performing ovulation (the release of eggs from the ovaries). Taking the pills can also reduce the heavy bleeding that she may experience during her period, can lessen the severe pain caused by menstrual cramps, and can cause her to have fewer periods and/or shorten the length of her periods. Heavy bleeding, killer cramps, and long periods are all symptoms of endometriosis. You know how excruciating and life-changing those symptoms can be. So if birth control pills can help reduce the symptoms, it's understandable why a woman would want to use them, and why her doctor would want her to use them.

With that said, I want to be very clear about what the pill does not do: it does not make endometriosis go away, and it does not prevent it from advancing over time. I know you've heard me say that repeatedly, but it's especially important to emphasize because I believe there are some doctors who think the pill can make endometriosis disappear. The pill may, in some women, be able to shrink an ovarian cyst, but it cannot be used in lieu of deep-excision surgery. It may slow down the growth of the endometriosis, but it does not stop it. The pill serves as a mask, suppressing the symptoms until a woman is ready to have surgery, or until she is old enough for her doctors to be certain she has endometriosis. The pill may not necessarily work for all women, but as a temporary treatment it can help many of them.

When I see or hear about an adolescent girl who is suffering through her first several periods with endometriosis symptoms, my initial reaction is that she should probably be put on the pill immediately. Her ovaries are in hormonal flux as they begin to "hatch" eggs. Taking the pill will suppress the increased effect of estrogen in the uterus and reduce those symptoms. The immediate reaction of some people may be "How can you suggest putting a thirteen-year-old girl on the pill?" But the purpose is not to prevent pregnancy, and her age is irrelevant. Whether she is thirteen or twenty-three or thirty-three, the purpose of prescribing the pill to a woman with symptoms of endometriosis is to diminish the symptoms so that she can go to school, hold down a job, maintain her relationships, and simply function in everyday life.

Birth control pills "totally worked" for Blaire, one of my patients. She started getting painful periods when she was seventeen. She went on the pill when she was eighteen and stayed on it for about thirteen years. "It became a necessity for me," she said. "When I went off my dad's insurance, I had a couple of months when I wasn't on the pill and the pain came back. I had to get back on the pill right away. My period while I was on the pill was very regular, very normal, very healthy. It began and ended when it should have, and it was very manageable."

When she reached her early thirties and was thinking about having children, Blaire decided to stop taking the pill. "That's when all hell broke loose," she said. "I think all those years the pill helped regulate the endometriosis, but it didn't stop it. It was still growing, just at a slower pace. When I got off the pill, it was like it was the endometriosis's time to shine. The gates of hell opened and little demons set up camp in my uterus. It was really, really bad."

Her doctor told her those were the cards she'd been dealt. "And my mom said I just had to deal with it." Blaire eventually became my patient, and I performed a three-and-a-half-hour surgery on her to clean out a very widespread case of the disease. She remains off the pill today and is pain-free. She and her husband are very excited to try to start a family.

"There is a stigma to being on birth control," Blaire said. "Some people have the misconception that you are sexually promiscuous or that there's a certain carelessness you have with your sex life when you are on birth control, when the reality is that it has absolutely nothing to do with sex. It's for pain management. You need it to function. You need it to live."

I introduced you earlier to Nicole, the psychologist who was diagnosed with endometriosis in her midtwenties (and who was told by a gastroenterologist to consider taking antidepressants). For the six years immediately following her diagnosis, she was on the pill, and it enabled her to accomplish what she wanted to accomplish during that time.

"I wasn't getting my cycle while I was on it, so there was less pain," Nicole said. "I was able to get my master's degree, finish my doctorate program, complete an internship, get married, go on my honeymoon, start my group practice. The pain emerged a few times a year, and it was horrific when it did, but it was better than suffering through it every month." Although the birth control worked to control her symptoms, the endometriosis was still building inside her the entire time. "I felt better while I was on the pill," she said, "but the damage to my body from the endometriosis was getting worse."

Kyung, an artist in New York City, was about twenty-four when she started developing very sharp pains in her lower abdomen. She had no idea what the problem was, so her friend, a cancer survivor, suggested that she keep a journal of her pain, recording when she got it, where she felt it, how severe it was, and how long it lasted. After a few months, Kyung realized the pain coincided with her period. She went to her OB/GYN, who did a laparoscopy and found endometriosis everywhere. But because the disease was spread so thin and because he knew his method of surgically removing it (with a laser) would have likely caused her considerably more pain, he decided to leave it alone and suggested instead that she take Lupron shots. Kyung, however, could not afford the shots because she had little money and no insurance, so she decided to try the doctor's alternative suggestion, which was to go on the pill in an attempt to suppress the symptoms for a while.

"I took it for two years to stop my period," Kyung said. "It served its purpose. It put the endometriosis pain to sleep. But it also caused me to gain weight, and it created mood swings. I took myself off it because I didn't like myself on it. I felt like I didn't have my head on right." The pill also didn't stop the endometriosis from growing. When her pain eventually returned, she went to a different OB/GYN, who found her right ovary to be almost triple in size because of a chocolate cyst. The doctor removed the cyst with a laser.

You will read more of Kyung's story later. I wanted to share this part of her story now, along with Blaire's and Nicole's, because they exemplify that the pill can do both good and bad. It can stop the pain, but it can also have side effects. It can help you get through the day for the time being, but it does not prevent the endometriosis from growing inside you.

What I also want you to take away from this chapter is that birth control pills are prescribed more commonly for reasons other than birth control. These circumstances include the attempt to regulate irregular periods, control menstrual cramps, and treat acne. Also understand that the pill does not cause fertility problems, as some people may believe—endometriosis does.

28

Pseudomenopause and Menopause

MENOPAUSE NORMALLY OCCURS IN A woman during her late forties or early fifties. It is defined as the time when a woman's ovaries cease functioning, thus ending the production of estrogen. Once she's in menopause, she will no longer have any menstrual periods and cannot get pregnant. Menopause is part of every woman's natural biology, though, through medication, her body can be tricked into it at an earlier age, an event known as medically induced menopause or pseudomenopause. Pseudomenopause, much like the pill, is recommended by some doctors to women with endometriosis to suppress the disease's symptoms, primarily the pain. Either by injection or in pill form, doctors prescribe the pregnancy hormone progesterone. I've had new patients tell me they have tried this option. For some of them, it doesn't work; the pain persists even during the pseudomenopause. For others, it affords some pain relief, but only for a short time. Many have told me that whether it worked or not was irrelevant because the numerous side effects were too much to handle.

A woman may undergo early menopause through a medication injected under the skin. Lupron is commonly prescribed for this purpose. Its primary mechanism is to suppress the production of estrogen. Since endometriosis feeds off estrogen, the idea is that the disease will no longer grow, and maybe even shrink, while the woman is in menopause. Like the pill, though, this alternative treatment serves as nothing more than a mask.

It's a short-term solution to the long-term problem of endometriosis. A woman who goes through pseudomenopause will feel many of the same effects that a woman who goes through natural menopause feels, such as hot flashes and extreme emotional highs and lows, to name a few. Lupron is not something I generally prescribe to my patients.

Jessica, whom you heard from in earlier chapters, went through several laser surgeries to treat her endometriosis. After three of those surgeries, she was put on Lupron for six months to prevent her from getting her periods while she healed. That means she went through menopause three times before age thirty-five.

"My mom's friend was going through menopause naturally," Jessica said, "and she was talking about her hot flashes. I said, 'I know, aren't they hell?' She couldn't believe someone so young was going through what she was going through. It worked, though, because it stopped me from getting my period each time, which would then stop the endometriosis pain. But I never felt very healthy on Lupron. I would break into sweats in dead winter when the temperature was below zero. I would sweat just driving to school. Looking back, I don't think I'd do it again. The next time I go into menopause will be the real time."

Monique, who shared her near-hysterectomy story, also took Lupron. Overall, it was not a good experience. She was on it for about six months in 2013 and a few more months in 2014 before undergoing surgery in early 2015. "It did help ease the endometriosis pain because I wasn't having my menstrual cycle," she said, "but it created all kinds of other problems. In 2013 I had hot flashes, night sweats, and literally the marrow in my bones hurt. I had no energy, it hurt to walk up the stairs, my joints hurt, and I had no desire to have sex or even be in a relationship with anyone. When I took it in 2014, I still had all those side effects, plus I was losing my hair and my memory was vanishing. I couldn't remember some of the simplest things."

Like any other medication, Lupron will work as prescribed for some women and not at all for others. Some may feel no side effects, and others may experience multiple ones. The fact that Monique tolerated roughly ten side effects for so long in exchange for avoiding the pain from her periods speaks volumes about the severity of the pain her periods were producing. But was it worth it? That's what each woman needs to decide.

If taking a drug like Lupron is ever presented as an option to you, please be very careful. If it makes your pain subside, that's good. But if you experience a lot of side effects, as some of my patients have described, you should probably reevaluate your situation and consider other alternatives. Mostly, however, remember that medically induced menopause, like the pill, does not make endometriosis go away.

Endometriosis may persist after menopause for two reasons. One reason concerns the fact that the body, particularly the fat tissue under the skin, continues to produce estrogen. Estrogen production stimulates the endometriosis foci. The second and more common reason is the excessive amounts of estrogen replacement therapy that many women use in order to ease the symptoms of menopause. Remember how certain endometriosis cases progressed with birth control pills in the pretense of masking symptoms? Similarly, there are many women whose endometriosis becomes worse while taking massive doses of estrogen replacement therapy.

Just recently, one of my patients needed emergency surgery due to massive internal bleeding at the age of sixty-two. The only explanation for this massive bleeding was a retrograde menstruation that could not escape through the cervix, but conveniently escaped into the peritoneal cavity. All of the excisions from her peritoneum tested positive for endometriosis. Although this is a particularly rare case of endometriosis, a patient who excessively uses estrogen replacement therapy is not treating her body the way it should be treated. Endometriosis patients who really need estrogen replacement therapy must understand that it may come with a heavy price.

29

Hysterectomy Not So Bad

YOU'VE READ ABOUT WHY A hysterectomy can be the wrong solution for a woman with endometriosis. Not only is there the possibility that it won't eliminate her pain because the disease could have already spread to other places, but its permanence means the woman can no longer have children. There are times, however, when it is necessary. My patients generally need hysterectomies only when adenomyosis has also developed. As I explained earlier, adenomyosis occurs when endometriosis cells develop in the muscle tissue of the uterus.

A hysterectomy for endometriosis is not an easy operation. The disease is often present where the anterior (front) rectum meets the posterior (back) cervix and vagina. Many surgeons avoid this area by doing a supracervical hysterectomy or an intrafascial hysterectomy. A supracervical hysterectomy removes the top half of the uterus while leaving the bottom half—the cervix—intact, even though endometriosis is almost always present in the bottom half. An intrafascial hysterectomy removes the cervix but leaves behind most of the surrounding endometriosis tissue and ligaments. When the vagina is closed, endometriosis remains at the top of the vagina. Even if the ovaries have been removed, this can cause painful sexual intercourse. Many doctors have a false notion that if the ovaries are removed, the body will no longer produce estrogen and, therefore, will not stimulate any remaining endometriosis, but that's incorrect. Estrogen can come from other sources, such as from the food you eat or from the body's fat stores. Endometriosis can even make its own estrogen. If a woman still feels pelvic pain after a hysterectomy, it's likely because the endometriosis is still present. This is why the first part of a hysterectomy operation for endometriosis, even if the ovaries are to be removed, should involve excising the endometriosis. Of course, if the endometriosis has been removed, there is no need to remove the ovaries. I believe that at least one ovary should be preserved during most endometriosis hysterectomies, especially if the endometriosis is excised before the hysterectomy.

In February 2015, I performed a hysterectomy on Carissa, the pediatric occupational therapist you met earlier (along with her husband, Drew). Carissa was just thirty-five years old, but she gladly welcomed my recommendation that I remove her uterus. She was about ten years old when she had her first period—an abnormally heavy and painful one, but normal according to all the women in her life who told her to suck it up. The pain from her periods intensified as she got older. Getting through college classes was difficult. She could no longer go to the beach or to the pool with friends or family during her period because her menstrual flow was so heavy. After having two children (a medical mystery considering how widespread her endometriosis was when she eventually came to me), she hurt too much to even play with them.

"It was really affecting my life," Carissa said. "In college, my gynecologist told me it was probably just stress, but it got worse and worse as the years went on. I always had to change the bed sheets. I had to carry a million pads with me everywhere I went."

Her gynecologist found a cyst in October 2014 and told her he could remove it. Carissa said it was supposed to be a twenty-minute surgery. "I was in there for two hours. When I came out, the doctor said endometriosis was on every organ," Carissa said. "After surgery, I felt worse than before I went in. He told me this was just the way it was going to be, and that he would do a hysterectomy in a couple of years. But I didn't think I could wait that long. I couldn't play with my kids. It was impacting my bowels. It was awful."

Carissa's sister-in-law was a patient of mine and recommended to Carissa that she meet with me. After looking at the results of Carissa's MRI, I had no doubt that she was a candidate for a hysterectomy.

"Dr. Seckin made sure that I didn't want to have any more children. He said a hysterectomy was a last resort for him, but I didn't want to live like this anymore."

I removed her uterus, cervix, and left ovary—everything except her right ovary—in a surgery that lasted close to seven hours. "When I came out of surgery, I felt amazing," she said. "The pain was instantly gone. I'm really a new woman now. All those years, I thought I knew what 'normal' was, but I had no idea. Since I'm so young, people tell me it must have been bad if I had a hysterectomy. Yeah, it was bad."

When a doctor tells you that a hysterectomy is the only way to end your pain, he or she may be right, but you need to ask a lot of questions first, especially if you still want to try to have children some day. Is a hysterectomy the only solution? Could the source of pain possibly be something besides the uterus, for instance the surrounding scar tissue on nearby organs? Does he or she do deep-excision surgery? Are there alternatives to a hysterectomy? If not, can your eggs be frozen if you would like them to be? If you choose to have a hysterectomy, what organs will he or she remove? Just the uterus? Part of the uterus? The cervix? The tubes? The ovaries? As I said, many doctors will only take out half of a woman's uterus. Some of them will leave the cervix because it's the most difficult reproductive organ to remove if it involves endometriosis; it's a risky and complicated surgery for doctors who do not regularly operate on endometriosis patients.

I've stated that one out of every fifteen or twenty patients who come to me has undergone a hysterectomy, and most of them probably weren't necessary. For those that were necessary, the women have come to my office either because the endometriosis has spread to other organs, or because the doctor who did the hysterectomy removed only some of their reproductive organs instead of removing everything necessary to eliminate the pain. Think of it this way: if a cardiologist tells a patient that three of her arteries are 99 percent blocked and she needs open-heart surgery, that surgeon is not going to go in and clean out just two of the arteries and leave the third one blocked. If a hysterectomy won't solve the problem you have with endometriosis because the disease remains in other parts of your body, then what is the point of having your uterus removed? If you decide to have a hysterectomy, be certain that it is a last resort, that you and your doctor agree on the definition of *hysterectomy*, and that there is no endometriosis anywhere else.

30

Freezing Your Eggs

SARA, A PATIENT I INTRODUCED you to earlier who said she would be "on the floor in a corner" without her pain medication, had endometriosis for about fifteen years before she was diagnosed. After having an ovary removed by another doctor in the summer of 2009, Sara came to me for surgery that fall.

"It was a four-and-a-half-hour surgery, and so much endometriosis was removed," Sara said. "I could not believe the previous doctor let me walk out of her office without telling me what was inside my body. My right ovary was basically dead, which it didn't have to be. I had severe endometriosis all over my uterine wall, which was giving me urinary tract infections. I was definitely in stage IV." Sara also had some endometriosis on her bowels, which I could not safely remove given its location, so I told her we might have to consider surgery again in a couple of years.

"Sure enough, about two years later, I had lost about fifteen pounds and knew something wasn't right," Sara said. "I thought this could be a result of the bowel issue Dr. Seckin had mentioned. He did a sonogram and MRI and found that the endometriosis in my bowel had spread quickly. He did another surgery and had to remove part of my bowel to get the endometriosis out. Then he had to reattach the bowel."

I told her after the second surgery that there was always a chance the endometriosis could resurface, especially considering how quickly it had spread between the first and second surgeries. I told her that if another surgery was necessary, a hysterectomy might have to be a consideration. She was in her early thirties with no children. I asked her if she wanted to have children; she said she didn't know, but she didn't want to rule it out. We talked about her options, including having her eggs frozen. She decided to do it.

Freezing Sara's eggs cost her thousands of dollars out of pocket. Her insurance didn't cover any part of the procedure, which is typical and something I would like to see changed in the future, but the cost didn't deter her from doing it. "If you think about it, we invest a lot of money in other things, like cars," she said. "Your body should be the most important thing you invest in. I was at a point where I didn't know if I wanted kids, but I did not want to let go of the option. I knew this disease could come back, and the next surgery could include a removal of everything."

Sara initially began the process of having her eggs frozen after my second surgery on her, but she decided it was too much for her body to handle right then. She restarted it in July 2014. "You begin by going in for a couple of appointments so they can get a sense of your cycle and determine when you should have hormone injections, and so you can take prenatal vitamins and get healthy," she said. The hormone shots, which contain high levels of estrogen, were injected in her abdomen area and caused her some nausea. The eggs grew very quickly. She then received a shot that released the eggs so they could be retrieved and frozen. The entire process was finished by August. "After your body has created all that space for the eggs, but the eggs aren't there anymore, you have a bloated feeling and are full of hormones, but during your next cycle it all comes out," Sara said.

The fertility specialists retrieved seven eggs, five of which were considered viable for freezing. They ideally like to retrieve many more than that, but considering that Sara had only one ovary, they were happy with what they were able to get.

If Sara decides she wants to have children, we would have to see if the endometriosis has resurfaced and estimate her chances of carrying a child to term. If the chances aren't good, or if we have to do a hysterectomy before she decides whether or not she wants children, she could have a surrogate carry the child using her eggs.

Sara said freezing her eggs has eliminated a lot of stress because she knows her eggs are safe no matter what the endometriosis may do to her in the future. It has also brought her some comfort when the issue of having children comes up. "When I used to go out with people and they asked if I wanted to have kids, I didn't know how to answer them because I didn't know if I could even have them. Now if I'm asked that question, I can answer it, and that's a relief for me."

If you aren't sure whether you want to freeze your eggs, you may want to consider the perspective of Dr. Avner Hershlag, chief of the North Shore-LIJ Center for Human Reproduction. He spoke about egg freezing at my 2013 medical conference. He related it to the biblical story in which Pharaoh had a dream and called upon Joseph for its interpretation. "If you remember, he dreamed about the seven fat cows and then the seven skinny cows," Dr. Hershlag said. "Joseph interpreted it that they were going to have seven fat years, when the crop would be great and they would be able to store up. And then, when they came to their skinny years, their years of famine, they would have this stored crop. If you think about it, egg freezing is like storing up for those later years when the ovaries are in famine."

The Care You Deserve

31

Your First Visit: What to Expect

MANY OF MY PATIENTS ARE referred to me by another patient who I've operated on, a friend or relative of theirs, by a gastroenterologist, urologist, or general gynecologist, or even occasionally by a cancer surgeon. Others find me online, through either my website, the EFA website, an independent business-review site, an interview with one of my previous patients, or a social-media site. Some of my new patients know about endometriosis when they first come to see me because of negative experiences they've had with previous surgeries. Others have never even heard the word. By the time our initial meeting is finished, they are usually confident that I can help them.

On average, women who come to see me have already undergone two to three surgeries by other doctors in an attempt to alleviate their pain, none of which worked for the long term. They have had one or both ovaries removed, a hysterectomy, an appendectomy, or a bowel resection (part of the small or large intestine removed). In other words, they often have been treated by surgeons who weren't even gynecologists, let alone endometriosis-surgery specialists. They were surgeons who weren't certain what the problem was but who thought it could be solved by removing part or all of an organ.

Many of my first-time patients have already seen multiple doctors, from general practitioners to gynecologists to specialists for diseases or conditions unrelated to endometriosis. The list becomes so long that when I ask them which other doctors they have seen, many have trouble remembering the entire list. These doctors often prescribed medications such as high-level painkillers, antidepressants, and others that negatively affected the women's moods and did nothing to treat what was really wrong. Knowing all this helps me connect immediately with a woman when she walks in the door, which helps her visualize and actualize a path toward healing.

At our first meeting, I don't initially have a pad of paper in front of me to write down everything she says. I don't have a pen in my hand. I just let her speak while I listen. It's an old-fashioned, face-to-face conversation. I give her as much time as she needs to tell me about the pain, the misdi-agnoses, the previous surgical experiences, and how her circumstance has affected her relationships, her work, her education, and/or her ability to be a mother. It's normally a very emotional meeting for her for several reasons, one of them being that it's probably the first time in years that someone has truly listened to her. She may shed tears while explaining what she's been through, get angry that nobody was ever able to help her, tell me more than once that she's at her wits' end. The most gut-wrenching part of her talk will concern the pain. She will describe it in ways that would make anyone else uncomfortable. One recent patient of mine, a physician herself, de-scribed her painful period as being like passing a bag of nails every month. Another patient, to describe the pain in her back, drew a picture for me of a snake-like creature with fangs. The patients always have similar symptoms, but they each have an original description of their pain that will at times give me goose bumps. That is when we begin to trust one another, and my work to make her better begins.

The next stage of our meeting is when I get out my pen and paper and take notes as I ask her specifics about her pain and her past attempts at treatment. The first question I ask is about her period. How painful is it? How old was she when the pain started? How long does it last? Does the pain surface before, during, and/or after her period? During ovula-tion? How heavy is the bleeding? Is it clotty? Has she taken any medi-cation for the pain? Does she have a disease she is aware of that could promote heavy bleeding? Anything she can tell me about her period will help me determine the best course of treatment.

I ask her if she has any gastrointestinal symptoms: gassiness, bloating, diarrhea, constipation. We then talk about sexual intercourse. If she is sexually active, I have to get more personal with my questions. It's a subject that's not easy for her to talk about, and I often have to ask her about it multiple times to get her to completely open up, but she eventually does because she knows by this point that I want to help her, that I probably *can* help her, and that the more she can tell me the better chance she will have of ending her years of misery. I ask if the sex is painful with deep contact, or if it hurts more in certain positions than in others. This type of information can give me a sense of which organs may be affected by endometriosis. It's also important to note that many of my patients aren't having intercourse when they come in, either because they are too young, they don't want to, or the pain is so unbearable they are afraid to try. All the questions I ask about intercourse relate to the physiology of the woman's body. I don't get too personal. For example, I don't ask if the pain causes relationship problems with her partner. If she wants to tell me about that, I'm certainly willing to listen, but I'm not going to force her to relive that emotional pain. It's not a detail that is going to help me find and excise the endometriosis. Besides, if she has a partner and the sex is painful, I can conclude that it is likely causing some problems without having to ask for specifics.

Our initial visit lasts about an hour—sometimes more, rarely less. It's a long meeting, but we're conducting a personal conversation that is necessary to have. Honestly, considering all the years the patient has probably been suffering with nobody willing to fully listen and understand her, an hour doesn't seem to me to be very long at all. And when I say an hour, I don't mean an hour that includes sitting in a waiting room to be called back, and then sitting in a small sterile room alone for several minutes waiting for me to come in. It's an hour of one-on-one face time in which she does most of the talking and I do most of the listening. The most important words that I say to her, at some point early in the meeting, are that I want her to trust me. Once that trust is established, she is on the road toward conquering this disease. From my perspective, it's a huge responsibility to be trusted to do work in someone's internal organs that she will never see but will only feel.

Her next visit is when I conduct a very thorough physical exam. If she did not bring someone with her during our first meeting—a partner, mother, sister—I highly recommend that she bring someone to the second. That person won't be in the examination room but will be in my office with us before and after the exam for support. She or he provides a second set of ears to hear everything I discuss with the patient, and to ask questions the patient may not think of.

During the exam, the first thing I do is examine her sitting up. I touch her back to see if she has any pain or tenderness, especially in the kidney area. I then have her lie flat on her back and pull her knees to her abdomen so that her abdomen is relaxed. I check her abdomen, liver, spleen, and any previous incisions. A lot of those incisions will tell me a story, depending on how long they are and where they are located. While I examine her, I ask her several questions: Do you have leg pain, or pain anywhere else? Do you have children? If so, were they conceived naturally or using in vitro fertilization? Have you had any miscarriages? Is there a history of cancer or endometriosis in the family? Are you on any medication? If so, what kind?

Following this, I conduct a gynecological exam with a female assistant in the room. Her feet go in the stirrups, and I engage her in casual conversation to help her relax her mind and body. I may ask if she is from the New York area and ask where she works, and then say, "By the way, I'm just examining your cervix to see if I can feel any abnormalities." I want her to know what I'm doing, but I also want to divert her attention from it as much as I can. We are dealing with a serious disease, and I am more than likely about to cause her some pain by touching the affected area. I touch her cervix with my finger, moving from right to left and from front to back. I then feel the ligaments on each side and can feel nodules if there are any. This is called a bimanual pelvic examination. Next, I ask her for permission to perform a rectal exam. This is called a rectovaginal examination. As I examine the rectum, I feel for nodules in the side walls. I then do a transvaginal sonogram, which shows me the ovaries and the uterine cavity. I look for polyps and fibroids that are inside the endometrial cavity and are the cause of heavy bleeding and clots. Then I carefully view the uterine muscle walls for the presence of adenomyosis and fibroids. Finally, I scan the ovaries for cysts, endometrioma, and adhesions. Again I evaluate the level of pain as the transducer is moved towards the cul-de-sac and pelvic sidewalls. If she feels and reacts with pain, I know that she very likely has endometriosis.

Next, we return to my office, and I explain to her where in her body I think the endometriosis is located, how serious it is, and what needs to be done about it. I draw some sketches on a board as I explain to her how the endometriosis has implanted on her internal organs. I show her slides and pictures to give her a better understanding of the disease. I explain that during surgery I will also look at other areas, such as her appendix and the rest of her bowels, to see if the endometriosis has spread to those parts.

If I think the patient is going to opt to have surgery with me, I follow up with a few more important steps. One is to send her for an MRI to further evaluate the tissues and look at the kidney system, and a CT scan to make sure I've covered every point in the body that I need to be concerned with. I also give her the option of consulting with a psychologist. As you well know from the patients' stories you've read, endometriosis can attack a woman mentally as much as it does physically. I feel it is my job not only to surgically remove all the endometriosis, but also to remove the negative psychological effects it causes. I believe psychological peace is an extremely important component of the overall health of my patients. While to a small extent I may have played the role of psychologist during our first meeting, I want each patient to have the opportunity to talk to a professional psychologist if she wants to speak more deeply about her pain, her fears, her relationships. It's a chance for her to get more comfortable before surgery and for me to make an even better connection with her.

I encourage patients to see a psychologist if they are depressed or if they are taking any medication that could affect their emotional well-being. For me, this is like ordering an MRI of their feelings and emotions. It is essential for me to see an evaluation of how they handle stress. The report I receive helps me build trust with the patient before surgery. Some of my patients have been counseled by Casey, a patient of mine whom you met in the chapter on nutrition. Casey is a social worker. She received several misdiagnoses from other doctors over many years and suffered four miscarriages. I have performed two surgeries on her, and she does a tremendous amount of work for me and in the community to spread awareness about endometriosis. She has worked on my blog and was head of the Westchester, New York, chapter of the Endo Warriors, which you will read about in the book's next section. As you can see in her following words, Casey can empathize with all my patients:

I'm there every step of the way with them if they want it, all the way through post-op. I encourage them to get excision surgery, and I try to calm any fears they have. This disease is pervasive; it affects relationships and friendships and career choices. Even with the best of care, these women have an altered quality of life. I help them with their self-esteem and make sure they understand that even though the disease impacts them, it doesn't define them. A lot of women worry about what they will find out when they wake up from surgery. They fear they may not even have endometriosis because so many doctors questioned them beforehand. They are worried that Dr. Seckin won't find anything and that they really might be crazy. Or, if he does find it, how bad will it be? Will they wake up without their ovaries? Will other organs have to be removed? There are so many what-ifs that make this difficult. I make sure they know that they are truly amazing and courageous, and that they are in the best hands.

The final thing I do is ask the patient to meet with other specialists on my team who may also be involved in the surgery. For example, if I think there are significant bowel lesions, I ask her to see my bowel specialist. If there may be kidney issues, I ask her to see my urologist. We will be 100 percent prepared going into the operating room with top-level expertise in every respect.

When all is said and done, my patient has had a minimum of three or four visits with me before surgery. I like to form a relationship with her. I want her to have an experience with me in the office. She should have the opportunity to digest our initial meeting and each subsequent one so she can ask any questions she may think of later that could help her make an informed decision. If she elects not to have surgery, that's certainly her prerogative. If she decides she wants the surgery, then we schedule it immediately. Once surgery is over, chances are very high that she will wake up a new woman, instantly feeling better than she has in many years.

The way I treat my patients isn't merely an example of how you can be treated, but of how you should be treated. Whether you are going to see your doctor about a minor ache or a major issue, you always deserve the best treatment.

Sara, who described freezing her eggs, probably developed endometriosis when she was about fifteen, but she wasn't diagnosed until she was twenty-nine, soon after getting sick during a night out. She had just arrived at a bachelorette party when she was suddenly hit with diarrhea and abdominal pain and nearly passed out. She somehow made it through the party and saw a doctor the next day.

"She barely greeted me, sent me for an ultrasound, and concluded that I had some cysts on my ovaries," Sara said. "She did surgery, removing the cysts and part of my right ovary, and she never came to see me after the surgery. They wanted me out of the hospital as soon as possible for some insurance reason. In fact, the nurses were trying to make me pee so they could get me out of there. I had never had surgery before, so I just assumed that was how surgery was supposed to go."

Sara went in a week later for her follow-up appointment:

The doctor told me that from what she saw during the surgery, I had a severe case of endometriosis. She told me that if I wanted to have kids, then I had to have them now, or else they wanted to put me on Lupron. It was just really weird the way she presented me with only these two options. I told her I didn't want to have kids now, and that I didn't want Lupron because I didn't even know what it was. She seemed to get angry that I refused both options, so she said, "Then I need to put you on birth control." I told her I had been on the pill before, and my body did not respond well to it. She said, "Then I don't know what to do with you," and she sent me home. She never really explained to me what endometriosis was, how severe it was, and where it had spread throughout my body. She just said that I had it, and if I didn't have kids now, then I wouldn't be able to have them at all. That was what I walked away with.

When Sara told me this story, I was thoroughly disturbed. Unfortunately, I hear stories like it too often. Please, if you ever walk away from a doctor who has treated you like that, keep walking. Find yourself a new doctor immediately.

Basira, who shared her case in the chapter on ovarian cysts, started getting symptoms of endometriosis, such as heavy periods and killer cramps, when she was eleven. She lived with them for more than a decade, assuming they were normal. When she was twenty-three, a sonogram showed she had a chocolate cyst on one of her ovaries. She also suffered back pain, leg pain, constipation, and painful intercourse. Basira did her research and was certain she had endometriosis.

"I wanted to make sure I found a good doctor, because I knew that not everyone could treat it," she said. "I did a lot of research on Dr. Seckin and heard really good things about him. When I went to him, I could tell he was an expert because he knew what to ask and what to look for. He wasn't just one of those doctors who said, 'I'll put you on birth control'—like my previous OB/GYN wanted to do. I knew I needed surgery, and so did he. Dr. Seckin didn't dismiss any of my concerns or my feelings about my condition. He took the time to assess my situation and figure out what was going on. He asked when I had begun menstruating and if I had painful periods, leg pain, painful intercourse. Being an obstetrician is a busy profession, and many of them just want to get you in and out, but not all women present the same symptoms. You need someone who is detail-oriented and can assess you the correct way."

Again, this isn't about me. It's about you receiving the proper care. Many doctors treat their patients with sensitivity, knowledge, and compassion, but you need to put forth the effort to find them. If you encounter a doctor like the one Sara had, trust your instincts and know that you deserve better.

32

The Gold Standard

LAPAROSCOPIC DEEP-EXCISION SURGERY IS WHAT I call the gold standard of endometriosis surgeries. By magnifying everything, laparoscopy offers a much clearer view. This allows me to perform surgery in the most precise manner possible. I have been modifying this surgical precision for years. My modification comes from enhancing an easier recognition of endometriosis by using the aqua blue contrast technique. This allows me to perform wide and deep excisional removal using cold scissors and to reconstructively repair involved organs, such as the ovaries, bowel, bladder, and ureter, with fine suturing.

It's a method I was introduced to more than twenty-five years ago after observing the works of Dr. Camran Nezhat and Dr. David Redwine, and while working alongside several surgeons in New York, including Dr. Harry Reich and Dr. C.Y. Liu, both prominent laparoscopic surgeons and pioneers in the field of endometriosis. At this time, only a handful of doctors perform laparoscopic deep-excision surgery for endometriosis, a deficiency I would like to see remedied. Learning and refining the procedure requires a great deal of experience, knowledge, time, precision, dexterity, and patience. And expertise in performing endometriosis surgery cannot be defined without the ability to treat unintended consequences —the complications.

What makes this surgery the most effective way to treat endometriosis is that it doesn't zap out the tip of the disease, as laser surgery does. Rather, it removes the inflammatory tissue down to its roots by bringing deep layers of the body into the surgeon's view. In this way, it relieves or even eliminates pain, and can possibly restore fertility. The surgeon not only removes diseased and damaged tissue but also skillfully reconstructs organs and restores their functionality. In terms of reconstruction, endometriosis surgery is like plastic surgery, except its aesthetics aren't visible the way a nose job is. The proof of successful reconstruction is pain relief for the patient after her organ function is restored. For this reason, it is imperative that every endometriosis surgeon have the ability to suture and tie tissues, and to return an organ to precisely where it should be. The organs must also function well after surgery. In sum, the skills required include not only the excision technique but also meticulous bleeding control, suture repair, and reconstruction and restoration of organs.

I describe this surgery to my patients using the analogy of an iceberg. Picture the peak of an iceberg (the endometriosis) protruding above the water (an organ in the body). Shaving off the top of the iceberg down to water level would appear to leave behind a clean and smooth surface. However, the largest and most dense portion of the iceberg remains below water. Even though it may not be visible, it's still there. That "shaving" would be analogous to endometriosis surgical techniques that use laser ablation, electrical fulguration, or some other procedure involving electrical current to zap the part of the endometriosis that is above the organ's surface. The portion below the surface is still there, left to continue growing and flourishing. Deep-excision surgery permanently removes the entire iceberg, or endometriosis nodule, and so provides the greatest amount of pain relief.

The way I perform the surgery follows a modified methodology and technique that I have trademarked. I follow the same sequence of steps in every surgery to enable me to remove the endometriosis as completely as possible. Some doctors start in different places each time or get sidetracked by something unexpected they find once they open up the patient. By following the same steps in a certain order each time, I feel more in control of and comfortable with what I am doing. If you switch procedures each time, you are more prone to miss something.

So how does the surgery work? A laparoscopy enables me to visualize the abdominal/pelvic region using an instrument known as a laparoscope. A laparoscope is a long, thin tube with a telescopic lens, multiple light sources, and a miniature video camera. A large monitor is set up across from me, on the other side of the patient, so I can clearly see everything inside her. The instruments I use are extensions of my hands, so my hands never actually enter the patient's body (they couldn't, given how small the incisions are). It's like having a set of chopsticks in each hand. As I watch the monitor, I move pixel by pixel to cut out every speck of the disease I can find using cold scissors. This is why dexterity and precision are so important. Organs are manipulated for viewing, biopsies are taken, the diagnosis of endometriosis is confirmed, and diseased tissue is removed. A surgery will last three to four hours on average, and sometimes up to five or ten hours. Given its difficulty, you can understand why so few surgeons have been trained, or want to take the time to be trained, to do this procedure.

The surgery begins with a small (approximately five to ten millimeters) incision made through the navel, into which a needle is inserted. For better visualization inside the abdominal cavity, carbon dioxide is injected into the abdomen. This colorless, odorless gas swells the cavity, lifting and separating the organs to allow the laparoscope to be safely inserted. Similar incisions will likely be made in the pubic hairline and/or over the ovaries, through which surgical instruments can be inserted.

Once all the instruments have been strategically inserted, I explore the organs and surrounding tissue, take biopsy samples, and then remove the endometriosis and adhesions. I begin with the colon, then I move to the ovaries, pelvic sidewall, uterus, and other organs. I inspect every inch of the abdominal and pelvic cavities, as well as the liver and diaphragm. Every abnormality I see in these areas may pertain to the woman's pain until proven otherwise.

One of the most critical aspects of excision surgery is the confirmation of the diagnosis of endometriosis by a pathologist, who views a sample of the removed tissue under a microscope. The pathologist reports to me the extent of inflammatory changes caused by the endometriosis, including whether any tissue may have been left behind. The pathologist will also determine if there are cancerous changes to the endometriosis cells. A recent study from Sweden suggests that patients with endometriosis who were treated with excision surgery had a reduced incidence of ovarian cancer compared with endometriosis patients who did not undergo the surgery.[xv] Similarly, controlled studies have proven that, compared to other methods, excision surgery offers the best outcome for pain relief and positive impact on quality of life. Whether we are treating something as significant as frozen pelvis or as small as a single peritoneal lesion, the gold standard is to excise without leaving any diseased tissue behind. Only the excision technique can treat for all symptoms of endometriosis, including painful periods, painful sexual intercourse, painful bowel movements, and leg and back pain during menstruation.

A patient's recovery period will vary. A woman who undergoes a three-hour surgery to have endometriosis removed from a small area will likely recover much more quickly than a woman who has an eight-hour surgery to remove it from several organs. My goal with every patient is to have her out of the hospital within twenty-four hours. I would rather have her moving and walking and getting her strength back in the comfort of her home than in a hospital, where she is in close proximity to other sick patients. If she is too sore to go home within a day, I won't force her to do so. Some of my patients have stayed as long as a week. It's longer than either of us would like, but if that's what she needs, then so be it. As for overall recovery time, I've had patients who went back to work in about a week and others who required a month or more. Every patient is different.

What happens if, after the surgery, the woman's pain doesn't subside as much as she or I expected? A small percentage of women I operate on will need to come back for another surgery, usually for one of two reasons: either the endometriosis was so deep that I could not get it all without risking the possibility of nerve damage, or I may have missed something because the length and complexity of the surgery caused what is known as surgeon's fatigue. If I could go for twelve or sixteen hours straight, I would, but it's just not possible. Nine or ten hours is about the maximum.

I never promise a patient that her pain will be reduced to a specific level; no doctor can guarantee a precise result with any treatment. In this way, too, every patient is different. Though many of my patients will tell you that I performed miracles on them (especially if they went through previous unsuccessful surgeries with other doctors), I don't perform miracles. There is no magic. I cannot control a woman's pain. What I can promise her going in is that I will remove each abnormal tissue separately, I will remove as much endometriosis as I possibly can, and I will not remove any of her organs unless it is absolutely necessary. I will also tell her that I have seen cases like hers before and that it is my goal with her case to have the same success as I did with the others. I video record each surgery from beginning to end. If a patient's pain comes back, together we will review the recording of the surgery step by step, and we will see what we can figure out.

A procedure with a high rate of success coupled with openness and honesty on the part of the surgeon—that's what every patient wants, whether she has endometriosis or another ailment.

NOTE: See image 16 in the photo section starting on page 93.

33

When Surgery Doesn't Go as Planned

I CLOSED THE LAST CHAPTER by describing deep-excision surgery as having a "high rate of success." Those are true words. Notice, however, that I didn't say a success rate of 100 percent. I treat each patient who comes to me as if her life depends on what I am able to do for her. People tend to think that successful surgery is a magical event, or that it is miraculous. There is no magic, no miracle. I do the absolute best I can with the tools I have. But my best doesn't always produce the perfect results we both want.

Nicoletta's painful periods started when she was eleven years old. Her story is similar to those of the other women you've read about: her family told her the pain was normal; she missed a lot of school and events because of the pain; she was told to deal with it by taking Advil or prescribed painkillers; she was misdiagnosed with IBS; she went to three OB/GYNs over several years who didn't know what to do for her; a fourth OB/GYN finally diagnosed her with endometriosis after she'd suffered for sixteen years; he attempted to treat her by using laser surgery; and she and her husband tried for five years to have children, with no success.

In 2011, after more than twenty years of suffering with the pain, Nicoletta found a doctor who specialized in treating endometriosis. "I was excited," Nicoletta said. "He said, 'I can help you with this, and you will be able to have children.'" Nicoletta scheduled surgery with him in

June. When she came out of surgery, she felt great. The surgeon told her that he had removed the disease.

"I really did feel amazing. I was so happy," she said. But the enjoyment was short-lived. The surgery he had done, like her previous one, was laser. "A month later I was in more pain than I'd ever been in," Nicoletta said. "I could barely walk. I limped into his office. He couldn't believe it. He just told me to go home, lie down, and take some painkillers. When that didn't help, I went back a couple of weeks later and had an ultrasound. He said everything looked perfectly fine and I shouldn't be having any problems. But there were problems. I told him I was afraid of getting my period next month. But he didn't know what else to do."

Nicoletta changed her diet and started seeing an acupuncturist, who recommended a couple endometriosis surgeons to her, one of whom was me. "I called both offices to get a feel for them, and I felt that Dr. Seckin's office was more professional and caring and on top of things," she said. "I met with Dr. Seckin in September 2011, and he questioned me in detail. He told me everything that I had been feeling without me having to say it. He immediately gave me hope."

I did surgery on Nicoletta in November 2011. The surgery lasted for eight hours. I did a resection of her rectum and placed stents in her ureters. I extracted twenty specimens that tested positive for endometriosis. This occurred just five months after her previous surgeon had told her that he'd removed it all and that everything on the ultrasound looked perfectly fine.

Here is the point in the story when I usually say that the patient lived happily ever after. But not this time.

"After surgery, my hemoglobin was low," Nicoletta said. "The nurses said I could stay in the hospital overnight, but I'm a nurse and figured I could take care of myself, so I told them I'd just go home. When I got home, I wasn't feeling well. I was very pale. Something wasn't right. By the third day, I felt that if I didn't go to the hospital, something bad was going to happen."

I was out of town after Nicoletta was discharged from the hospital, so I wasn't there when she came back in, but a couple of other doctors on my team were there to take care of her. They found that she had some internal bleeding, and she was also in a lot of pain. They gave her three units of blood and monitored her until she felt good enough to go home. But two days later she was back, and severely sick. She vomited several times on her way to the hospital.

"I honestly thought I was going to die," Nicoletta said. "It turned out that the stitches on my rectum had opened up, and I'd become septic. I had to see several infection-control doctors. It was determined that I needed to have a colostomy." A colostomy is a surgical procedure that brings the healthy end of the large intestine out through an opening (stoma) made in the abdominal wall. Stools moving through the intestine drain through the stoma into a bag attached to the abdomen. A colostomy is usually prescribed to give the colon a chance to heal after a trauma such as surgery or cancer. It can be temporary or permanent.

Nicoletta's nightmare continued. "I had the bag for four months, and my weight dropped all the way down to eighty-three pounds. I had to go on disability and almost lost my job. It was really bad," she said. "I was in the hospital for probably fifteen days while they tried to figure out what bacteria were invading my body so they could get the antibiotics right. At one point, I didn't eat for twelve days."

When I returned to New York, I met with Nicoletta and her husband. To say I felt horrible about what had happened doesn't come close to describing my devastation. Although she had every right to be angry at me, believe it or not she had the opposite reaction. Even though I knew I had done my best in surgery, I felt undeserving of the compassion Nicoletta showed me considering everything she'd been through.

"Oh, don't get me wrong. I was mad," Nicoletta said. "I was angry that this happened. I was angry that Dr. Seckin was gone when it happened. I wouldn't be human if I didn't feel that way. But when I met with him, he apologized, and I could tell he was on the verge of tears. I knew how sincere he was. That's when a calmness came over me. I realized the doctors from his team who were there to take care of me did just that. One of them visited me in my room every single day. The internal bleeding was something that could happen in any surgery, and they took care of it. As far as my becoming septic, I knew that wasn't negligence. It wasn't a mistake he made. Sometimes things like that can happen, especially when you consider how bad the endometriosis was and that the surgery took eight hours."

Fortunately, there was a "happily ever after" ending to Nicolette's story. Despite all the complications, the excision surgery worked in more ways than one. After the colostomy (which was successfully reversed), not only was she able to begin living a relatively pain-free life for the first time since she was a child, but a year after her surgery she became pregnant. She gave birth to a healthy boy in August 2013. The following year she got pregnant again, and she gave birth to a healthy girl in April 2015. In both cases, the babies were conceived without the use of in vitro fertilization.

"I believe there is a reason for everything," Nicoletta said. "I know others may have gone a different route and stayed angry with Dr. Seckin, but I decided to take the view that I was no longer in pain, and I was meant to go through everything I went through in order to one day have these beautiful children."

Though Nicoletta's surgery didn't go as planned, I wanted to share it with you to show you the reality of this line of work, and to remind you that doctors are human. No surgery is "routine." There's certainly nothing routine about surgery for endometriosis. I have had cases in which, even after the most meticulous excision surgery, I had to reoperate. In some cases the lesions were hidden so deep that I didn't see them. In others the endometriosis was so aggressive that new lesions formed soon after the initial surgery. Each surgery requires extreme focus, precision, and 100 percent effort, but even then not everything always goes according to plan. A story like Nicoletta's is extremely rare among my patients. It is my goal, no matter how complicated a patient's case may be, to make sure it stays that way.

34

New Lives (Literally) after Surgery

YOU JUST READ ABOUT THE two new lives Nicoletta and her husband created after she had deep-excision surgery. Let me share with you a couple more. Kyung, the artist from New York City whom I introduced to you in the chapter on the effects of birth control pills, came to me for surgery in February 2013. It was a four-hour surgery in which I removed eighteen lesions and her appendix, along with a lot of scar tissue from a laser surgery she'd undergone with a previous doctor. In my notes following her operation, I wrote, "Chance of getting pregnant is almost fully removed or significantly diminished." The endometriosis had done a lot of damage to her reproductive organs. "Significantly diminished," though, means there is still hope, and certainly more hope than she'd had before the surgery. I suggested to her that if she wanted to try to get pregnant, she should try very soon.

"My fiancé and I followed his advice and tried to get pregnant right away after the surgery, but nothing happened," Kyung said. "In December, I started to feel some pain again. I went to Dr. Seckin, and that's when he dropped a bomb on me: that I had adenomyosis"—endometriosis cells that have invaded the muscle tissue of the uterus. "He told me that I might need to have a hysterectomy at some point. It was a total shock to us. I'd had the endometriosis surgery hoping that everything would be fixed and that we'd be able to get pregnant, and now it appeared that wasn't going to happen. We cried. We pretty much mourned for a month."

Kyung had no idea that the emotional roller coaster she'd been on that year—ranging from a successful surgery after years of pain to the development of adenomyosis ten months later—was just beginning. In April 2014, knowing that a hysterectomy might be in her near future, she got pregnant. Sadly, however, the baby did not survive.

"You first hear the heartbeat at the seven-week ultrasound," Kyung said. "I didn't hear it. They told us the baby had stopped developing after about five weeks. When I went in to see Dr. Seckin, he told me it was a really good sign that I was able to get pregnant at all. That's not necessarily what you want to hear when you are going through a miscarriage, but I understood what he was saying. It gave us hope."

Kyung and her fiancé got married and traveled to Puerto Rico for their honeymoon. "I actually took my ovulation kit with me," Kyung said. "I was ovulating then, and we wanted to try to get pregnant. We had stopped trying for several months so that we could clear our minds and focus on the wedding." When they returned from their honeymoon Kyung took a pregnancy test, and it was negative. But just days later, when she should have had her period, she didn't. She took another test, and it was positive.

"I was so excited. I took the test at about 5 a.m., but thought it was too early to wake my husband up. I just kept looking at the stick. I couldn't believe it. Finally, at 6:30, I woke him up and showed it to him." Her husband was very happy, but he cautioned Kyung not to get too excited considering all they had been through. Kyung went to her OB/GYN, who confirmed that she was pregnant.

"We scheduled the seven-week ultrasound for Christmas Eve," Kyung said. "We were so nervous because we knew it was going to make or break our Christmas. Thank goodness we heard the heartbeat! We were both crying. It was the best Christmas gift ever. The doctor told me that I was still at high risk because of the endometriosis and the previous miscarriage. I couldn't exercise or do anything during the first trimester. But by the second trimester, everything was looking good." Kyung's baby boy was born in July 2015 and entered the world healthy, weighing just under nine pounds. There were no complications, and Kyung and her husband are very happy parents.

You also read earlier about Nicole, the psychologist. Nicole was diagnosed with endometriosis during a laparoscopy when she was in her

midtwenties. The disease had created a major blockage in her right ureter, reducing her kidney function. Doctors inserted a stent into the ureter
to open it, and they also burned off some of the endometriosis with a
laser. After the surgery Nicole was told that she was "as good as new."
But she wasn't.

You may recall that Nicole went on the pill for six years following her
diagnosis. That gave her some pain relief, but the endometriosis continued
to grow. Roughly every six months for those six years and beyond, she had
to have the stent in her ureter replaced to avoid infection. She also underwent four surgeries in which doctors burned more endometriosis.

When Nicole stopped taking birth control so that she and her husband could try to have a baby, the pain was vicious. She eventually got
pregnant, but she miscarried. She became pregnant again a year later and
this time gave birth to a healthy baby girl. That was the wonderful news.
But some bad news came with it. During her pregnancy, doctors could
not insert a new stent in her ureter. As a result, her kidney function decreased to just 12 percent.

"It was recommended that I have a nephrectomy [surgical removal of the kidney] and a hysterectomy," Nicole said. But she had a
major issue with that advice. "My husband and I wanted to have
another child."

Starting soon after their daughter was born, and after Nicole refused to have the nephrectomy and hysterectomy, she and her husband tried to have another child. As she describes it, it was eighteen
months of hell:

> I gradually developed new symptoms that I brought to the attention of my fer-
> tility specialist. I began to have numbness in my leg, accompanied with pain-
> ful cramps. The specialist said that I "must have lifted something heavy," and
> he referred me to my primary-care physician and a neurologist. I researched
> the symptoms on my own and found that they may have been related to my en-
> dometriosis since the pain came and left with my menstrual cycle, but nobody
> listened to me. My primary-care physician prescribed muscle relaxers and
> pain medication. The pain and numbness were debilitating; I could barely
> walk when they were at their worst, let alone drive or function at work. I
> could barely sleep. I reduced my days at work because of the illness. I was also

experiencing frequent bowel movements, which became very painful as time progressed. I returned to my fertility specialist, and he referred me to a gastroenterologist because he thought I may have a "bowel disease." I continued to blame my endometriosis, but my opinion and the research that I presented were dismissed.

After those eighteen months, and with no pregnancy, her symptoms worsened.

"The pain did not abate after my menstrual cycle, like it usually did. It remained throughout the entire month," Nicole said. "I resumed taking birth control pills and contacted my doctors, who sent me for several tests, such as CT scans and MRIs. All the test results were negative. I was prescribed pain medication because just eating was causing severe pain; the endometriosis was on my colon. But if I didn't eat, I felt faint. I lost twenty pounds within a few months." It was about that time that she drove herself to the emergency room—where the gastroenterologist told her that antidepressants might be helpful.

Nicole took matters into her own hands and searched for an endometriosis specialist. That's when she found me, late in the fall of 2010. "Dr. Seckin said that I was among his top ten patients who had intricate problems due to endometriosis," Nicole said. "It was in stage IV. It was causing nerve problems in my leg. It had attached to my rectum. It had built up on my pelvic wall, and I also had fibroids and a hernia. He said I may need to have both a ureter and colon resection."

The surgery lasted eight hours. Despite the horrible condition she was in, I was fortunately able to excise the endometriosis without removing any organs. That was in February 2011. Nicole was back to work in March, had another stent inserted in her ureter in April, and started in vitro shots in June. And the best news of all? "I was pregnant in July," Nicole said. She had her second healthy daughter in early 2012.

As wonderful as Kyung's and Nicole's stories are, I am glad to say that I see positive cases like theirs quite often, as I'm sure many surgeons who perform deep-excision surgery do. Just as endometriosis can cause infertility, removing it can often have the reverse effect, depending on how serious the case is. Several of my patients who had given up hope of ever having children are mothers today. This is why deep-excision surgery is so effective, why laser surgery is not, and why reproductive organs that have endometriosis on them should be removed only as a last resort—not for the sake of the surgeon's convenience or because of his or her lack of knowledge about what is really wrong with the patient.

35

Laser Surgery and Electrosurgery

AS I STATED IN LAUREN'S story in the first chapter, any mention in this book about the use of laser surgery to treat endometriosis lesions refers to the "burning off" method, which involves using a high-energy heat source. You've met several patients of mine who underwent this type of surgery with previous doctors, resulting in numerous complications, including higher levels of pain. This doesn't mean that a laser cannot be effectively used during surgery to treat endometriosis. Let me explain the bad and the good. This will get a little bit technical, but I will try to state it in simple terminology. My goal is to educate you in case your doctor ever suggests laser surgery to treat your endometriosis.

Surgeons use two types of electrical current: coagulation current and cutting current. Coagulation current is high energy, or high voltage, and should not be used to try to remove endometriosis. It is difficult to control and lacks precision. It will burn the lesion on the surface (remember the iceberg analogy?) and some of the surrounding tissue, accelerating the pathology of the disease. And what will result? Endometriosis causes pain because of the scarring it creates. Scarring pulls the tissue, making it hard and thick. When a surgeon burns the endometriosis with a high-energy laser, it causes that tissue to adhere more deeply to the underlying tissue. The result is an inflammation on top of the endometriosis-causing inflammation, giving you two layers of inflammation. The already-hard tissue becomes even more tense and more scarred, and continues to further bury the endometriosis (the core of the disease) that lies underneath it. Not only does burning the endometriosis fail to rid the patient of the pain she's been in, it will likely cause more pain. She may enjoy a brief reprieve immediately after the surgery (though that isn't always the case, as Lauren can testify), but over the long term her symptoms will likely become worse than they were before the surgery. If she eventually decides to undergo deep-excision surgery, her laser surgeon has made the procedure more difficult for me or whoever performs it.

I want to be clear that coagulation using bipolar cutting current can be used during endometriosis surgery to stop minor bleeding. That's a common and acceptable use for coagulation, and it's something I do. But using coagulation to try to remove endometriosis and using it to stop bleeding are two completely different things.

If deep-excision surgery is not an option for you, and your choices are to have a high-energy laser surgery or to try some other short-term remedy, be it a nutrition regimen or acupuncture or medication, I would choose the "other short-term remedy" without hesitation. In my opinion, using a high-energy laser is nothing more than a convenient, sexy tool that superficially sprays light energy and changes the color of the endometriosis tissue. It's like a video-game gun that gives doctors the license to indiscriminately shoot the tips of the icebergs. It kills good tissue around those tips and creates scar tissue. It temporarily solves one problem, but it creates others. I would say six out of every ten patients who come to me have undergone some type of high-energy laser or electrical surgery at least once or twice. Jessica, a patient I introduced you to in the chapters on neuropathy and menopause, had so many laser surgeries that she cannot remember the exact number.

"I was diagnosed with endometriosis when I was twenty-one. The doctor said I was covered in it," Jessica said. "She burned it out, but I had to keep having another surgery and another one, year after year. In the twelve years I went to her, I probably had eight or nine laser surgeries. She finally told me that it was growing back so fast each time that I needed someone with more training to help me. She said she had a friend in New York City; it was Dr. Seckin." I had to do two surgeries on Jessica in fifteen months because the endometriosis and the scarring from the laser surgeries were so bad. Today, she is able to live a normal, relatively pain-free life.

Laura, who shared the compelling story about her ectopic pregnancy, endured six laser surgeries in about ten years before she found me to perform surgery on her the way it should have been done to begin with:

> *Every year I'd go in and they would clean it out. I'd be okay the first three or four months; then it would start to hurt again. After a year, it was back in full force. Unfortunately, laser surgery was the only thing that helped. I wasn't really thinking of the dynamics of surgery and taking into account that having a lot of surgeries was not good for my body. And I knew nothing about the effects of laser surgery. It became like clockwork for me. I could schedule each surgery a year in advance. The doctor who did those surgeries did fine for what he was doing, and he had the best intentions, but he just wasn't knowledgeable enough about the disease. He was named one of the best in New Jersey. That shows you how little people know about endometriosis. When I hear someone with endometriosis say they had surgery but still don't feel well, I say, "Let me guess, you had laser surgery." And they did.*

Unlike techniques using shotgun laser, cutting current is low voltage and, like the carbon-dioxide laser, can effectively excise endometriosis lesions. The heat generated is confined to vaporizing water-containing cells that the surgeon sees; it doesn't affect normal tissue located deeper. Keep in mind that there are various kinds of laser that should be avoided. Some terms you may hear are Argon, KTP, and YAG. Only carbon-dioxide laser surgery is precise—so precise that it vaporizes water in cells with a minimal surrounding thermal effect. The carbon-dioxide laser is a great instrument and, when used at the junction of diseased tissue and normal tissue, can result in an accurate dissection, the same as cold scissors. However, it leaves behind some burned tissue and, more importantly, is not always safe when used on the rectum, ureter, or large blood vessels. For me, nothing beats cold scissors, but carbon-dioxide laser is an option.

The lesson here is that unless your doctor says he or she is going to excise your endometriosis using a low-voltage cutting current or carbon-dioxide laser, stay away from laser surgery. Most surgeons who say they are going to use laser surgery to treat your endometriosis are referring to the burning method. Don't get me wrong: there are very skilled surgeons who use the burning method (as Laura said, her doctor was named one of the best in New Jersey), but it doesn't matter how skilled that surgeon is; he or she can't win using a method to treat endometriosis that requires cutting with high-voltage heat, because the field left behind will always be a cooked field. He or she is trying to get rid of an inflammation with a burn, which is an inflammation itself. We need to use surgery that does not promote inflammation.

When I look at tissue that's been burned by laser surgery, I find carbon deposits in it. When I do surgery, I sometimes feel like a detective going into a house that's been torched. How do fire investigators find where the fire started? Because they are trained. They know. And what they find is never anything good.

NOTE: See images 14 and 15 in the photo section starting on page 93.

36

Robotic Surgery

SINCE 1975, SIGNIFICANT PIONEERS HAVE pushed forward the frontiers of minimally invasive surgery (vaginal surgery, hysteroscopic surgery, and laparoscopic surgery), and I applaud the development of another minimally invasive technique: robotic-assisted surgery, usually referred to simply as robotic surgery. But not only are there no substitutes for deep-excision surgery, as I've stated throughout this book, there are also no substitutes for how I do that surgery—not even robotic surgery.

A study published in the *Journal for Healthcare Quality* in 2011 by researchers from Johns Hopkins University[xvi] found that promotional materials about robotic surgery listed on hospital websites generally overstated the benefits of the surgery, ignored the associated risks, and may have been influenced by manufacturers. Findings from the study also suggested that hospitals were "allowing industry to speak on behalf of hospitals and make unsubstantiated claims," and that there was an inherent conflict of interest in using manufacturers' materials on hospital websites.

The study observed that from 2007 to 2011, the use of robots to perform various common procedures had increased by 400 percent. An estimated 41 percent of US hospital websites advertised robotic surgery, and of those that did, 89 percent touted its clinical superiority over conventional surgery. But the websites' claims about robotic surgery went much further:

- 85 percent claimed it brings less pain.
- 86 percent claimed it produces a shorter recovery period.
- 80 percent claimed it causes less scarring.
- 78 percent claimed it causes less blood loss.
- 32 percent claimed it improves cancer outcomes.

However, none of the websites that highlighted robotic surgery explained its potential risks.

The *Medical Daily* reported in the summer of 2015 that a retrospective study of fourteen years of FDA records on robotic surgery conducted at Cornell University found that "out of 10,624 [adverse] events, there were 144 deaths, 1,391 injuries, and 8,061 device malfunctions."[xvii] The authors concluded that "a nonnegligible number of technical difficulties and complications are still being experienced during [robotic] procedures," despite widespread implementation of the technique.

In 2013, Dr. James Breeden, president of the American Congress of Obstetricians and Gynecologists, issued the following statement: "While there may be some advantages to the use of robotics in complex hysterectomies, especially for cancer operations that require extensive surgery and removal of lymph nodes, studies have shown that adding this expensive technology for routine surgical care does not improve patient outcomes." Consequently, Breeden continued, "there [are] no good data proving that robotic hysterectomy is even as good as—let alone better than—existing, and far less costly, minimally invasive alternatives."[xviii]

When surgeons with limited laparoscopic experience use a robot, it may appear to them that the robot is superior. That's because they did not achieve proficiency in the procedures before using the robot. Many robotic programs were started by gynecologic oncologists who know open abdominal anatomy but lack the skills necessary for using straight laparoscopic instruments. Despite the scarcity of supportive data, robotic surgery has been rapidly adopted into gynecologic practice, and its use has grown at a rate far exceeding that of laparoscopy. This growth results from gynecologists who, unlike general surgeons, fail to learn proper techniques for performing cost-effective laparoscopy with reusable instruments.

A couple of things are clear. Robotic surgery requires larger and more incisions than conventional laparoscopic surgery, and robotic surgery for endometriosis does not use palpation, a necessity to feel rectovaginal disease. An endometriosis surgeon should not rely on robotic surgery for a better outcome. A better outcome cannot be achieved when the surgeon sits fifteen feet away from the patient, when several large incisions are made, and when instruments cannot be changed as quickly as they should for bleeding control. Granted, there is a steep learning curve for traditional laparoscopic surgery, and the introduction of robotic laparoscopic surgery has increased the percentage of patients who undergo a minimally invasive approach. But robotic surgery doesn't offer better ergonomics, increased dexterity, or improved visualization. It is simply easier for a surgeon to learn to perform it.

37

A Possible Link to Ovarian Cancer

I'VE STATED THAT ONE OF the most critical aspects of excision surgery is the confirmation of the diagnosis of endometriosis by a pathologist looking at a tissue sample under a microscope. The pathologist will also determine if cancer is present. Without this important step, Angela, a patient of mine from Mississippi, would probably still not know that she had cancer. Angela endured a barrage of endometriosis symptoms as a teenager: painful periods, killer cramps, heavy bleeding, fatigue, and painful bowel movements. When she was fifteen she underwent a CT scan, which revealed cysts on her ovaries. Her doctor told her they were nothing to be concerned about, so she didn't let them worry her. But as the years went on, the symptoms worsened.

When she was in her early twenties, Angela and her husband researched her symptoms and felt confident that she had endometriosis. She convinced her gynecologist to do exploratory surgery. What was supposed to be a thirty-minute procedure took three hours. "She said it was the worst case of endometriosis that she'd ever seen," Angela said. "She burned it all with a laser, and my symptoms only got worse after that. She wanted me to go on Lupron, but I had done my research and knew that wasn't the way to go."

Angela called multiple endometriosis surgeons across the country, from California to New York, and she finally selected me. Five months after her surgery, I performed a five-hour deep-excision surgery, including a bowel resection, on her. As I do following all surgeries, I sent her biopsies to the pathologist. What came back was shocking to both of us: Angela had ovarian cancer originating from endometriosis. Cancerous changes occur at the nucleus of the cell and can only be diagnosed under microscope. I sent the biopsy out for a second opinion, and the cancer was confirmed. It was an exceptionally slow-growing cancer. "The CT scan that showed the cancerous tumors on my ovaries matched up perfectly with the CT scan that showed the cysts when I was fifteen, the ones the doctor said I didn't have to worry about," Angela said. "In other words, the cancer was there when I was fifteen."

The second pathologist who confirmed the cancer, a gynecologic oncologist, performed a hysterectomy and appendectomy on Angela three months after I did my surgery. The cancer was estrogen-fed, so after surgery Angela was put on a drug that removed all estrogen and progesterone from her body. She is still on that drug today, has regular CT scans and blood work, and is doing well, with no signs of cancer.

Any doctor who performs deep-excision surgery and sends biopsies to a pathologist could have discovered the cancer I did, but few surgeons take those steps. Angela's previous gynecologist simply burned the surface of the diseased tissue and missed both the extensive bowel disease, and the ovarian cancer. Angela continued to have severe symptoms because the disease, located in her bowel, was never diagnosed. Neither was her ovarian cancer. As I noted earlier, a Swedish study[xix] suggests that patients with endometriosis who are treated with excision surgery had a reduced incidence of ovarian cancer compared with endometriosis patients who did not have excision surgery. This information put the role of endometriosis at the center of controversies involving ovarian cancer, the deadliest female disease. That's why, in my practice, I strongly advise patients with endometriosis to have their ovaries removed after menopause if they have ovarian cancer in their family. I have long believed that endometriosis can cause ovarian cancer. I don't see the cancer every day; probably one in every five hundred surgeries I've done has revealed its presence. But the American Cancer Society estimated that more than twenty-one thousand new cases of ovarian cancer would be diagnosed in 2015, and that more than fourteen thousand women in the United States would die from the illness.[xx] When you couple those numbers with the number of undiagnosed or misdiagnosed cases of endometriosis every year, I expect that we will one day learn there is a clear link between endometriosis and ovarian cancer.

Support:
Now and in the Future

38

The EFA

THE ENDOMETRIOSIS FOUNDATION OF AMERICA is a public health advocacy organization founded on four pillars: awareness, education, research, and effective intervention. I formed it with the support of several of my patients, and it was brought into the public eye in 2009 when Padma Lakshmi joined me as the cofounder. My vision for the EFA has been to bring awareness to endometriosis in the same way former first lady Betty Ford did for breast cancer. The subject of breast cancer was taboo before Mrs. Ford started discussing it. The five-year relative survival rate for female invasive breast cancer patients in the United States has improved from 75 percent in the mid-1970s to 90 percent today,[xxi] due primarily to heightened awareness, early detection, and better treatments. Padma realized the powerful impact sharing her endometriosis battle could have for the millions of women around the world suffering with the disease, and she didn't hesitate to join me in my mission. Every March or April, the EFA holds a weekend conference on endometriosis to educate the medical community including doctors, researchers, other medical experts, and medical students. It draws a higher number of attendees from all over the world than any other endometriosis conference in the United States. Our discussion topics include the latest techniques and technologies in surgery, diagnostic methods, nutrition and whole patient care, research, and policy.

We cover new aspects of endometriosis that will get the medical community absorbed in and engaged with the latest possibilities in tackling the disease. But it's not just a conference for medical professionals - it's for you, too. Because the conference gathers the foremost endometriosis thinkers from around the world, we invite the public to meet them and have their questions answered on day three, which we call "Awareness Day." This free event is dedicated to those who have the disease or who know someone who has it. Experts weigh in on topics ranging from postmenopausal disease, fertility and pregnancy, quality of life impact, and disease heredity. In 2015, Awareness Day attracted about 150 people, our largest turnout ever. The weekend concludes with our annual fundraising gala, the Blossom Ball, which brings in numerous pop culture celebrities who support the EFA's efforts. Throughout the rest of the year, the EFA works hard to educate the public by distributing informational pamphlets and posters, and by visiting schools to educate students through our rapidly growing and very successful EN-POWR Project, which you will read about in the next chapter. You will also read in subsequent chapters about how we target future doctors with our education efforts, and how we put a big focus on research with the hope of one day finding a permanent cure. The Blossom Ball receives a lot of attention because of the celebrities who support it. It's an extremely important event because the money it raises funds our education efforts. But it's those education efforts that we really want people to know about. Through our education initiative, we visit schools, businesses, community organizations, and the like to inform students, employees, and volunteers about endometriosis. Every week, we take phone calls and answer e-mails from our office about the disease. When awareness about endometriosis reaches the level where it needs to be—that is, on par with breast cancer or the like—it will be because of the grassroots efforts of this staff. The EFA is here to help you, but it also needs you to help spread the word. We've been at this for just six years, and we are off to a very good start. Please help us keep that momentum rolling.

39

ENPOWRing
the Young Generation

THE BEST WAY TO SPREAD awareness about something is by word of mouth. It may take some time to build momentum, but if the message is important and effective, people will tell other people until it resembles a snowball rolling down the side of a mountain, getting larger and larger at an unstoppable speed. That's what is happening right now with the EFA's ENPOWR Project. ENPOWR, which stands for ENdometriosis: Promoting Outreach and Wide Recognition, was started in 2013 as part of the New York State Department of Health's Teen Health Awareness Campaign. It is the only school- and community-based endometriosis-education project of its kind in the United States. We visit schools, summer camps, community programs—wherever there's a need—and give an interactive presentation that explains what endometriosis is, how to recognize its symptoms early, and how it can be treated. To promote early diagnosis and intervention and improve the current ten-year average delay to diagnosis in the United States, ENPOWR targets teenagers aged fourteen and above. We also educate school nurses, teachers, administrators, and parents through the program. We would like to reach anyone who's interested in learning more about the disease and who can help us spread the word about it. Thanks in large part to New York State Senator Jeffrey D. Klein, the project has received a state government grant each year for the last three years.

By the end of 2015, The ENPOWR Project had educated more than 10,400 male and female adolescents through 443 presentations across New York City, Long Island, Westchester, Binghamton, Ithaca, Rochester, Albany, and Syracuse. We have four full-time employees dedicated to the initiative's implementation, part-time health educators, and several volunteers and interns who make the program successful. Still in its pilot phase, ENPOWR has exceeded our expectations in such a short time. While we continue to learn and execute best practices, we are now developing a model that will allow ENPOWR to reach adolescents throughout the entire country. This is not a sex-education course. It's training about reproductive health that describes normal and abnormal symptoms with respect to pain, women's menstrual periods, and how to monitor and be an advocate for one's health. Presentations are designed for a co-ed audience. In fact, we often find that our most challenging questions come from boys who have seen their mothers in a lot of pain with horrible cramps. These kids care. If you provide them with knowledge, they will soak up that information and initiate positive change. The presentation can be life-changing for many of the girls in our audience. One sixteen-year-old girl wrote to us afterward: "I learned that I may have the disease and that my long periods and heavy cramps may not be normal. I shouldn't have to miss school for this." A living-environment teacher at a school in Upper Manhattan told us the following after our presentation: "As I was leaving the school this evening, one of the students approached me and told me she felt her doctor thought her painful discomfort was normal and she would grow out of it. But now she feels she should see a specialist. She was going to listen to her body and take control." And then there was this extremely gratifying remark from a health teacher at a high school in Albany, New York: "One of our students was not going to be able to graduate because she had too many absences. After she heard your presentation, she was diagnosed with endometriosis. Her absences were excused as a result, and she will be graduating on time in June!"

One of the most telling pieces of data we get at our presentations comes from the pre- and post-tests we give to each audience member. The survey contains several questions about endometriosis, including what it is, symptoms, diagnosis, timing of disease onset, when and how to seek treatment, and options for treatment. Among all students to whom we had given the test through early 2015, the average percentage of questions they answered correctly in the pre-test was 30.7 percent. In the post-test, their scores jumped to an average of 90.7 percent. This statistic indicates just how little most young people know about the disease, but how well they can understand it once they are given some information. When the presentation is finished, we encourage the audience to "take the pledge" and share everything they learned about endometriosis with family and friends. Out of the numerous important facts and statistics to remember about this disease, probably the most important one is that most women who have it are not diagnosed until they've had it for at least a decade. This is why it is so important for us to reach these kids when they're kids. The more they know now, the better chance they have of detecting the disease early, which could make all the difference in their lives—in their health, their relationships, their education, their job opportunities, their ability to have children, and their overall happiness.

40

Educating Doctors

I INITIALLY PLANNED TO WRITE a book that would have been more about the science of endometriosis, which probably would have made my target audience doctors and future doctors. I intend to do it one day. But after talking with my colleagues and my many patients who wanted to be part of this project, I realized that the best way to bring more awareness to the disease would be to first reach the women who have it or who think they may have it. Getting through to doctors is not easy. Some are open to new ideas and to learning new techniques. Others boast the attitude that they've been through enough years of medical school and have practiced long enough to know all there is to know. That's why nearly all the women who have shared their stories with you, and why most women who come into my office, were misdiagnosed, treated for a condition they didn't have, or even told that their pain was a fabrication of their minds by other doctors.

Our foundation regularly distributes literature to doctors' offices and clinics. I travel across the United States and abroad giving lectures and teaching the art and science of endometriosis surgery. We send e-mail blasts to gynecologists about the best ways to treat the disease. We hope that our efforts are working. But one of the best ways for us to reach other doctors is through you. It's a challenge to get and hold a doctor's attention; I know, because I'm one of them. From the stories you've read, you know that some doctors don't even listen to their patients. But since doctors' days are filled with patients walking through their doors with various ailments, I think the chances are pretty good that if anybody can get through to them, it might be a patient.

Besides using this book to learn about what is happening in your body, please use your newfound knowledge to educate your doctor while you advocate for yourself. You can increase your chances of receiving the treatment you deserve while you potentially help the next patient who comes in with killer cramps, fatigue, leg pain, or any of the other symptoms of endometriosis.

Hundreds of healthcare professionals have attended our medical conferences over the last five years—MDs, PhDs, researchers, and residents in training. At each conference we talk about the new techniques, debate issues about the disease, and award a scholarship to an attendee who is currently doing his or her residency. Our medical conference topics have been: "From Stem Cells to Radical Excision Surgery" (2010), "Let's Talk About Sex & Endometriosis…Seriously!" (2011), "Tapping the Roots for the Next Generation" (2012), "The American Perspective" (2013), "Politics, Ethics and Controversies" (2014), and "Ending Endometriosis Starts at the Beginning" (2015). But we need to go much deeper. Do you know that most medical schools and residency programs do not include endometriosis in their curriculum? It's not mandated.

Think about that. A disease that causes you or your loved one excruciating pain every day, that alters the way you live your life, that messes with your psyche, that causes you to miss large chunks of work or school, that negatively affects your friendships and your partnership isn't required to be discussed in medical schools. Are you insulted? I am. I work hard to educate doctors and the general public about the importance of recognizing deep-excision surgery as the gold standard of treatment for this disease, yet many people don't even know how to pronounce the word *endometriosis*. This must change, and I am doing everything I can by working with legislators and educators to get the subject mandated as part of medical-school curricula. A doctor can't diagnose somebody with something that he or she knows nothing about. With an estimated 176 million women worldwide afflicted by the disease, every person graduating from medical school should have a thorough understanding of what endometriosis is, how to recognize it early, what causes it to be confused with other problems, and the proper way to treat it.

If you are in residency or are considering the medical field as a potential career, this is a moment to implement serious and necessary change. We need to have qualified doctors ready to diagnose and treat them when the disease surfaces. If you are a medical student, or want to pursue medicine, recall the stories my patients have shared about their visits to doctors who didn't know what the disease was, didn't know how to properly treat it, didn't know whom to refer them to, told them it was no big deal, removed organs that didn't have to be removed, or called them crazy and sent them home. Do not become one of those doctors. Become a doctor who listens to his or her patients with empathy and believes their stories. Embrace awareness of this disease, and learn everything about it that you can. The more you know, the more lives you will save—even if you do so indirectly by referring patients to a qualified doctor who can help them. And the more you know, the more your patients will trust you, which will only help them and you.

41

A Cure

IS THERE A CURE FOR endometriosis? My colleague, Dr. Reich, thinks so. He has never viewed endometriosis as a chronic disease throughout his thirty years of excising it.

"If endometriosis came back every month, there would be no point in doing surgery," he says. "The endometriosis cells in many women have been around since birth. These cells begin a cycle of chronic inflammation on a monthly basis starting with menstrual periods. Fibromuscular tissue is deposited around the endometriosis glands and connective tissue with resulting pain. If diagnosed early, this tissue can be excised completely using the laparoscope. If diagnosed late, the same is true but requires a more complex surgery. Unfortunately, this type of surgery sometimes may include bowel resection and resection of small portions of the upper vagina behind the cervix. Most of these cases can be diagnosed by a simple rectovaginal exam in the doctor's office. MRI is rarely indicated. Assisted reproductive techniques should not be necessary for these women to conceive after laparoscopic excision."

Continuing with Dr. Reich's opinions: "Many fears of patients are based on the ideas that the disease will always worsen and recur, and that the risk of recurrence is supposed to be very high. In fact, no clinical data exists to determine whether endometriosis is a progressive and/or a recurrent disease, and many recurrent clinical symptoms may be explained by inadequate response to medical treatments and/or incomplete surgical excision of the disease."

He believes that true recurrence of the disease is rare. In most cases, the surgical excision patient does not get much worse after the initial surgical excision diagnosis. "Clinical recurrences" can often be explained by incomplete or inappropriate treatments. Most recurrences occur in areas involved during the initial surgical procedure. A study of second-look laparoscopy showed that recurrent disease occurs most frequently at the site of the treated disease after surgical treatment of early endometriosis, reflecting incomplete excision or ablation of the disease. After treatment of colorectal endometriosis, most re-operated patients are treated in the same area, suggesting that part of the disease was left behind due to an inadequate surgical procedure or because some organs were undertreated to minimize the risk of postoperative complications.[xxii] Using the term "cure" in relation to endometriosis is complicated. If, following excision surgery, a patient regains her quality of life with the elimination of pain, never requires pain medication, and is able to have one or more children, should we say she is cured? Or should we instead say that she has been treated successfully? No matter what terminology we use, the only thing that matters to me is that, after excision surgery, patients are able to live their lives the way they want to live them.

With that said, endometriosis is probably the least-researched subject in women's health care in the United States, which is why the EFA is heavily involved in facilitating groundbreaking research for finding a genetic component to the disease. The EFA has funded small studies at Johns Hopkins Hospital, but our most significant funding has gone to the ROSE Study. The ROSE (Research Outsmarts Endometriosis) Study, in partnership with Lenox Hill Hospital and the Feinstein Institute for Medical Research at North Shore-LIJ Health System, established the first endometriosis tissue bank. The ROSE Study has three main research goals: to develop early diagnostics for endometriosis, especially in adolescents; to comprehensively define the genetic components underlying the disease; and to develop new laboratory assessments and mouse models of endometriosis to test new approaches to preventing the disease. A very powerful five-minute video on the ROSE Study can be found at www. endofound.org/rose-study. As is stated in the video, "This is a disease that we can understand. It just has not had the kind of sustained attention in terms of basic research that many other common diseases have."

Still, despite the ongoing research, and despite the fact that the disease is highly treatable under experienced and skilled surgeons, I want to be very clear: we are many years, maybe decades, away from finding the genetic component that can lead us to a cure or to a method of prevention. Look at all the diseases we have been working on for the last half century or more for which we still don't have a cure. Once we identify the genetic component of endometriosis, we will be able to focus on finding a treatment without surgery. Everything worthwhile takes time. This is definitely worthwhile, and it is going to take time.

It is clear that even among endometriosis experts, controversy over disease etiology remains. The need for answers founded in evidence through research is essential.

42

Support Groups

KYUNG, WHO SHARED HER STORY about becoming pregnant after surgery, is a relatively quiet person by nature, but she has been one of my more vocal patients when it comes to spreading awareness about endometriosis. After Kyung and I set a date for her surgery, I invited her to attend a dinner party that I hosted for about fifty of my patients, some of whom had been with me for more than a decade. It is something I do every now and then to create and maintain a community among my patients so they can support each other and future patients.

Just days before the party, I was scheduled to give a presentation at Harvard University, but a snowstorm canceled the trip. I decided to show my presentation at the party. "Seeing that presentation before the surgery really helped," Kyung said. "It inspired me to later start an online journal about my battle with the disease."

Several of the women in the room, and some of their husbands, bravely stood up and shared their stories of fighting the disease. After several of them spoke, Kyung had the courage to tell her story. "I'm shy in front of crowds, but I felt compelled to share my story with them," Kyung said. "Every woman in that room had gone through surgery, and I was about to. I wanted them to know how I felt and how nervous I was. I got very emotional. But they all said, 'You'll be fine.' After I spoke, several of them came up to me and showed me the scars on their abdomens. I had never met an endometriosis patient before that, and now I had all these women who had gone through what I was about to go through on my side. It was a good feeling."

A handful of groups exist to spread awareness about endometriosis and to provide support to those who have the disease. Endometriosis.org is an international support group that I highly recommend. This group is administered by Lone Hummelshoj, who has been vital to raising awareness and conducting research on the disease. She has also worked tirelessly to implement legislative changes in the European parliament concerning the care for endometriosis. Debra Bush, who is incredibly experienced with managing endometriosis support groups, heads another support group, focusing mainly on adolescent awareness in New Zealand. Her stupendous efforts, spanning decades, encouraged me to start the high school education program with the EFA.

Another notable support group is HysterSisters (www.hystersisters. com). The organization provides hysterectomy support (not just for endometriosis patients) from "diagnosis to surgery through recovery and beyond." Its website offers various resources, including articles and a support forum. According to the website, the group covers "pre-op, post-op, gynecologic treatment options, surgical procedures, fibroids, endometriosis, menopause, hormonal issues, pelvic floor, GYN cancer, oophorectomy, sexual dysfunction, and a step-by-step guide through the weeks before and after hysterectomy."

Another group I recommend is the Endo Warriors (www.endowarriorssupport.com). Founded by three endometriosis patients, the group provides resources and sponsors online discussion forums. It also matches patients with volunteer "endo buddies," who will meet with patients face to face. It has chapters in New York, New Jersey, and Colorado and hopes to expand into other states.

Please contact these groups if you are interested in joining one of them, if you need emotional support, or if you have questions. They exist to help people like you, and they have been great resources for many of my patients.

43

Finding the Right Doctor

THROUGHOUT THIS BOOK I'VE EMPHASIZED that if you think you have endometriosis, it is crucial that you find the right specialist, and as soon as possible, to receive the proper treatment. Finding the right doctor is not an easy process, but hopefully you can learn from the stories of my patients and avoid the pitfalls they encountered.

Begin your search for an endometriosis specialist by reviewing your symptoms with your family doctor or another trusted medical professional. Ask them to assist you with recommendations, referrals, and follow-up care. Throughout the process, bear in mind the challenges some of my patients went through; learning from their experiences may help you determine if a doctor is the right one for you. Maintain very high standards when selecting your doctor. Endometriosis is a serious health issue that deserves only the best treatment.

Above all else, your endometriosis specialist should know everything there is to know about the disease. Keep in mind that most gynecologists who perform endometriosis surgery are not necessarily specialists. They will likely prescribe medications to suppress your ovaries, but the endometriosis will remain after the medication is stopped. They may also perform laparoscopy to diagnose endometriosis, but they will not carry out the necessary excision. One of the reasons for this incomplete approach is the fear of creating complications or risks—endometriosis, after all, often involves multiple organs and the depth of the lesion cannot be anticipated until it is completely excised. You need to find a specialist who has exceptional surgical skills and training, access to the most modern surgical equipment and techniques, a current understanding of various treatments, and an openness to complementary approaches. There are many competent specialists who practice according to these principles.

PREPARING YOURSELF FOR AN APPOINTMENT

- Before seeing a specialist, it is important to gather as much information about your symptoms as possible, as well as your medical history.
- If you have medical records from previous physicians, take them to the appointment, especially operative reports and pathology reports from surgical procedures.
- Complete the "Consider Endometriosis" survey and the "Personal Pain Profile" and take them to your appointment. These worksheets, available on the Endometriosis Foundation of America website (see "Resources" at the end of the book), will help you speak with your doctor about the symptoms you're experiencing.
- Think about other ways to describe your symptoms, concerns, and fears. Be specific. How much pain do you have on an average day, and how often? Is there a time of day when the pain is worse? Does the pain come and go? What helps alleviate it? How upsetting and disruptive is it? Do specific activities trigger it? Does it interfere with your daily activities or personal routine? Does pain accompany bowel movements? If you're sexually active, does deep penetration increase the pain? And, most important, is the pain worse on one side than the other?
- Don't be afraid to ask questions.

WHAT TO CONSIDER WHEN SEEKING A SPECIALIST

- Does the doctor specialize in both medical and surgical treatment of endometriosis?
- What percentage of his or her patients are young women and girls?
- Does the doctor have experience with related conditions?
- What is the doctor's attitude about your role in your health care? Is he or she willing to receive input from you?

- Does the doctor allow ample time for thorough conversation and examination, or does he or she rush through your appointment?
- Is the doctor able to explain surgical procedures and treatment options clearly and in terms you can understand?
- What are the doctor's beliefs about different hormone therapies (oral contraceptives, IUD, etc.)? Can the doctor discuss his or her reasons for prescribing certain medications, as well as the associated pros and cons?
- What does your intuition say? Are you comfortable speaking with the doctor? Does he or she listen to, acknowledge, and address your concerns? This must be someone you can trust and talk to openly.
- Does the doctor work cooperatively with other specialists who have a history of caring for endometriosis patients (e.g., GI doctors, pediatric gynecologists, psychotherapists, etc.)?

What to Consider When Discussing Treatment Options

- Discuss the specifics of the examination the doctor performed. Were the uterus and the ovaries mobile? Was the uterus anterior toward the abdominal wall or posterior toward the rectum? Was either ovary stuck to the pelvic sidewall? Was the rectum stuck to the cervix? Were any nodules felt during the rectal examination?
- Always ask about all available treatment/management options—surgical and medical—and choose the approach you feel most comfortable with and that is best suited to your lifestyle.
- When discussing medications, ask the doctor to explain exactly what each one is for. For instance, is it for pain relief or hormonal suppression? Also ask about risks, side effects, and drug interactions. Be certain to understand the duration of intended treatment, and schedule follow-up appointments to monitor results.

What to Consider When Discussing Surgical Treatment

- How does the doctor plan to use surgery to treat endometriosis? Does he or she specialize in laparoscopy? Does he or she plan to use laser (burn) or surgically excise (cut out) the endometriosis tissue?
- Will your surgery be documented with images? Will it be video recorded?
- How clearly is the surgeon able to explain the procedure? What exactly will be done during the surgery? For example, will endometriosis be

removed, or will it be an exploratory (look-only) surgery? Why? Most women should be wary of a procedure for diagnosis only. The surgeon should have the capability to complete the procedure properly (i.e., excise the disease).

- Is the surgeon openly discussing complications and risks? Is he or she experienced to treat complications?
- Is the doctor affiliated with a hospital that regularly treats endometriosis? Is there a dedicated operating room with dedicated personnel associated with the surgeon? Does the facility have a team of surgeons established to address different elements of surgical treatment? Will your surgeon have other experienced surgeons (general, colorectal, urological, etc.) in the operating room with him or her?
- What can be expected after surgery? How much pain can you expect? How can you lessen the pain? What are post-op restrictions for returning to school, work, exercise, other activities, and your normal routine? Learn how you can help to prepare yourself and your body for the surgery.
- Be sure to ask your doctor's office for a pre-op and post-op routine to assist in your healing process.
- Never rule out obtaining a second opinion. Or a third. Or more!

44

Insurance

IN TODAY'S WORLD OF SKYROCKETING health-care costs, the treatment people seek isn't always based on what they need, but rather on what they can afford or what their insurance covers. Most insurance companies have strict guidelines they follow when deciding whether or not to cover a procedure. Sadly, the guidelines don't cover much when it comes to endometriosis-excision surgery. Many insurance companies will pay for the "peeking in" part of the procedure—the laparoscopy—but they do not consider the excision, or actual removal, of the disease to be treatment. This is because most insurance companies conveniently consider the surgery to be experimental or investigational. They do not recognize the value of endometriosis excision surgeries, and instead ignore the fact that the surgery is necessary. For that reason, many doctors who do complex, time-consuming operations such as deep-excision surgery to remove endometriosis do not accept insurance. This is where things have to change with insurance companies, and increased awareness will make a difference.

For a surgeon to be reimbursed by insurance, the surgeon must submit operative and pathology reports to the insurance company. Several months after the insurance company reviews the reports, the surgeon may be paid. While a doctor should be fairly compensated, a patient's financial situation should not get in the way of her receiving the treatment she needs.

I am not contracted with any insurance company, but I do take out-of-network insurance. That means in order for me to be able to work with your insurance company, the company would have to allow you to go out of network. The same applies to any surgeon who is not contracted with an insurance company. If you have out-of-network benefits, it should be listed on your insurance card. But don't rely on that. Call your carrier and make sure you are covered.

You have read some of Monique's story. Monique, a government employee, can only make changes to her insurance in November of each year. Those changes go into effect two months later, in January. When Monique decided in mid-2014 that she wanted to have surgery with me, she found out that her insurance would not cover any of the surgery, so in November she switched insurance coverage to a carrier that would cover half the cost. The new insurance kicked in two months later, and I did surgery the following month, in February 2015. Getting coverage for the procedure took some creativity and patience on her part, but she saved a lot of money by doing the research to figure out her best option and by waiting to have surgery until that best option was available to her.

If your insurance company does not allow you to go out of network, do not give up hope. It will take some time and effort, but you can make your case to your carrier for why they should make an exception and let you see the surgeon you have chosen. You can tell them how many doctors you've been to within the network who didn't know how to treat endometriosis, how many unsuccessful surgeries you've had, and why the doctor you have chosen can do the surgery that you need to have done. You will need to prove to the carrier that you have done everything possible within the network, and with no success. The doctor can also support your effort by sending a letter to your insurance company requesting that an exception be made. The letter will describe the surgery he or she does and why it is the best option. To me, it's common sense. Why would an insurance company want to continue paying for unsuccessful surgery after unsuccessful surgery performed by doctors within a network when a doctor outside the network can solve the problem? But common sense isn't always used in situations like this, which is why you need to present your case to your carrier with as much detail and evidence as you can. When you are seeking an endometriosis-excision surgeon, know your insurance coverage as well as or better than your insurance company does. Ask questions, and if something doesn't sound right, ask again. You need to have a direct relationship with your insurance company and not be afraid to ask them questions. And never be shy about calling them more than once. This is your health, and you are your own advocate.

If you do not have insurance, cannot go out of network, or cannot afford to pay for your treatment, you can apply for a low-cost medical loan. Most practices have staff that can put you in touch with an appropriate lender. You may recall that my patient Kyung was a self-employed artist with no insurance. She secured a loan to pay for her surgery. Although borrowing money for medical treatment isn't ideal for anyone, it was an investment in Kyung's health and her future, and it paid off. She not only was able to move forward in her career, but also was able to get pregnant, something she (and I) thought would likely never happen.

"It's been worth the cost," Kyung said. "Knowing that you have a cyst that could burst is frightening. And cleaning out the endometriosis is necessary because the pain is not something you want to live with. I think it's just a reality that endometriosis patients have to deal with."

As you search for a surgeon who can do the proper surgery while you take steps to make sure you can pay for it, do not panic and rush into surgery. Yes, I have patients in such debilitating pain that the surgery should be done as soon as possible. Yes, you want to have surgery as soon as you can so the disease doesn't continue to spread and make your life worse than it already is. But with that said, a surgeon well trained in deep-excision surgery will be able to remove the disease from your body, whether it's tomorrow or months from now. If Monique had rushed into her surgery before her new insurance started, it would have cost her twice the amount she paid. She had to endure the pain for a little longer than she wanted, but she managed to do it and saved a lot of money in the process. Be leery of surgeons who tell you that surgery must be done immediately. Don't let them talk you into believing that the disease will rapidly progress to the point where nobody can fix it. A deep-excision-surgery specialist can fix it, no matter what stage it's in or how severe it is. Get it done as soon as you can, especially if the disease is in an advanced stage, but first make sure you have done your homework on the financial part.

The financial side of endometriosis has to change in order for women to receive the treatment they deserve. I continue to work with legislators and those in the medical community to advocate change, but more help is needed. You need to contact your elected officials and tell them your story. Tell them about the disease, what you have been through, what insurance issues you faced, and how much the disease has cost you—and not just in dollars. Your conversation with them may be the first time they've ever heard the term *endometriosis*. Teach them, and bring the sense of urgency to battling this disease that it deserves. The more awareness we bring to endometriosis, the more doctors who treat it the way it should be treated, and the more insurance companies that recognize it as the devastating disease it is, the better chance we have of making the proper treatment more affordable soon for the millions of women who are suffering.

Epilogue

JUST DAYS BEFORE THE MANUSCRIPT for this book was due to my publisher, and with everything written except the epilogue, I received some of the best news from my patient Laura that a doctor could hope for. I'm sure you recall Laura's frustrations in trying to deal with her endometriosis: the OB/GYN who told her that her pain was a "woman issue" that she had to learn to deal with; the numerous laser surgeries she endured; the ectopic pregnancy that resulted in a miscarriage and nearly the loss of her life. Laura said she felt "95 percent sure" she couldn't have a child because she only had part of one ovary remaining, and it didn't function well. I probably would have assessed her chances at less than that, but after her surgery that small chance remained. And in June 2015 Laura miraculously gave birth to a healthy baby girl.

Her pregnancy was high risk, so her doctor monitored her closely. "I made it through the magic twelve-week mark, and I was evaluated each month after that," Laura said. "The baby remained healthy and continued to grow. It was a very uncomfortable pregnancy because as the baby and my belly grew, it put a lot of strain on the scar tissue I had from all the surgeries, but I wasn't complaining. As long as my baby was healthy, I was happy."

After I removed Laura's endometriosis, she got a tattoo on her wrist that says *Vivi La Vita*—"Live Life" in Italian. "It's become a security feature for me," Laura said. "Anytime I have a bad day, I look at it and remember that I can finally live life." Every woman deserves to have that security. She should not be forced to have her life dictated by a dreaded disease.

I had two objectives in writing this book and in asking my patients to share their stories: for you or your loved one to get healthy, and for all of us to create a worldwide awareness about endometriosis. I hope that I have taught you enough about the disease that you will be able to recognize if you or someone you know may have it. Know the symptoms. Know the potential misdiagnoses. Know that the pain is real. Know that your doctor may have very little knowledge about the disease. Know how much the disease can affect relationships and work. Know the importance and responsibility of educating adolescent girls and boys about it. Know that it can affect fertility. Know how it should be properly treated. Know what questions to ask your doctor. Know that a hysterectomy should only be a final option. Know that you or your loved one is not crazy. Know how the disease can alter the course of a person's life. Be your own advocate. Stand up for yourself. Demand the proper treatment.

For centuries, other ailments have been blamed for the havoc caused by endometriosis. It's time to end the disease's anonymity, expose it to the world, and put an end to the destruction it creates. Talk about endometriosis to everyone you know. Pass this book on to a friend, and encourage that friend to pass it on to someone else. Give it to your doctor and start a discussion about it. Talk about the disease on social media. If you have endometriosis and are comfortable publicly discussing your condition, offer to write about it or to be interviewed for an Internet site, a newspaper, or a magazine. Join an endometriosis support group, or start your own. If you're a parent, tell administrators at your child's school about our ENPOWR Project, and help us get into the school to educate the students and staff. If you are in medical school and haven't learned about this disease and the proper way to treat it, encourage your school to make it part of the curriculum.

REMEMBER THE STATISTICS:
- An estimated 176 million women worldwide have endometriosis.
- At least 10 percent of American women of childbearing age have endometriosis.
- Diagnosing endometriosis takes an average of eight to twelve years.

- Early detection and timely intervention are vital to the prevention of pain, suffering, and infertility.
- Endometriosis is a treatable disease.
- Surgical excision–the gold standard–is the best treatment for endometriosis.

Enough is enough. Please take care of yourself first, then help me raise awareness about this disease. *Vivi la vita!*

Resources

THE FOLLOWING LINKS CAN BE found at the website for the Endometriosis Foundation of America: www.endofound.org. You are welcome to download free copies of any of this outreach and education material. Check the website often as materials are updated regularly.

Also visit the website for my surgical practice, www.drseckin.com, for more information on endometriosis and the work I do.

For more information about endometriosis, visit www.endofound.org/disease-information-and-support.

For resources, including printable brochures, fact sheets, symptom tracking tools, posters, and EFA logos, visit www.endofound.org/resource-materials.

For more information on the ENPOWR Project, visit www.endofound.org/the-enpowr-project.

For more information on the EFA's educational events and medical conference, visit www.endofound.org/medicalconference.

Acknowledgments

As an endometriosis surgeon, I could never successfully do what I do without the committed team of knowledgeable and passionate people around me. I've learned the same is true when it comes to writing a book about this disease. Thank you to the countless people who have helped me throughout my career and to those who have helped make this book a reality. The board and staff at the Endometriosis Foundation of America, your work moves mountains.

Padma Lakshmi, thank you for your vision, courage, altruism, and voice in helping me combat this disease.

Harry Reich, your pioneering work has not only inspired me, but thousands of surgeons around the world. Mina, the irreplaceable family writer who helped me with this book, thank you. And my wife, Elif, for your tireless support, encouragement, and unparalleled, eternal friendship – I would not be able to do any of this without you.

Bill Croyle, thank you. Without your work this book would not exist.

Thank you Jeanne Rebillard, Jon O'Neal, Sallie Sarrel, Selma Rondon, and Thom Graves.

Finally, I want to thank all the brave women and men who shared their stories that brought this book to life: Angela, Annie Rose, Basira, Beth, Blaire, Carissa, Casey, Diana, Elisa, Elissa, Eve, Jessica, Julie,

Kyung, Laura, Lauren, Liza, Michele, Monique, Nicole, Nicoletta, Sara, Stephanie, Rupi Kaur, Tom, and Drew.

Endnotes

[i] Endometriosis.org, "Facts about endometriosis," http://endometriosis.org/resources/articles/facts-about-endometriosis/.

[ii] *Journal of Endometriosis and Pelvic Pain Disorders,* G. David Adamson, Stephen Kennedy, Lone Hummelshoj, "Creating solutions in endometriosis: global collaboration through the World Endometriosis Research Foundation," 29 March 2010, http://www.j-endometriosis.com/article/creating-solutions-in-endometriosis--global-collaboration-through-the-world-endometriosis-research-foundation-art006549.

[iii] *Human Reproduction,* Hadfield R, Mardon H, Barlow D, Kennedy S., "Delay in the diagnosis of endometriosis: a survey of women from the USA and the UK," 11 April 1996, http://www.ncbi.nlm.nih.gov/pubmed/8671344.

[iv] *Endometriosis: A Guide for Patients,* The American Society for Reproductive Medicine, 2012, http://www.asrm.org/uploadedFiles/ASRM_Content/Resources/Patient_Resources/Fact_Sheets_and_Info_Booklets/endometriosis.pdf.

[v] *Human Reproduction,* S. Simoens, L. Hummelshoj, and T. D'Hooghe, "Endometriosis: cost estimates and methodological perspective," 2007, http://humupd.oxfordjournals.org/content/13/4/395.full.pdf.

[vi] *Journal of Pediatric & Adolescent Gynecology,* P.A. Suvitie, MD, M.K. Hallamaa, MD, J.M. Matomäki, MSc, J.I. Mäkinen, Prof., and A.H. Perheentupa, MD, PhD, "Prevalence of Pain Symptoms Suggestive of Endometriosis Among Finnish Adolescent Girls (TEENMAPS study)," 10 July 2015, http://wwwjpagonline.org/article/S1083-3188(15)00261-2/abstract.

[vii] *Journal of Fertility and Sterility,* Camran Nezhat, M.D., Farr Nezhat, M.D., and Ceana Nezhat, M.D., "Endometriosis: ancient disease, ancient treatments," 2012, http://www.endmarch.org/wp-content/uploads/2014/09/Endometriosis-Article.pdf.

[viii] *New York Times,* Associated Press, "House Approves Eliminating 'Lunatic' from Federal Law," 5 December 2012, http://www.endofound.org/endometriosis-ancient-disease-ancient-treatments.

[ix] *Journal of Fertility and Sterility,* Camran Nezhat, M.D., Farr Nezhat, M.D., and Ceana Nezhat, M.D., "Endometriosis: ancient disease, ancient treatments," 2012, http://www.endmarch.org/wp-content/uploads/2014/09/Endometriosis-Article.pdf.

[x] Endometriosis Foundation of America Medical Conference 2015, Dr. Sawsan As-Sanie, "Pain mechanisms in endometriosis: understanding the neurobiology of chronic pain to enhance patient care," April 2015, http://www.endofound.org/video/sawsan-suzie-as-sanie-pain-mechanisms-in-endometriosis-understanding-the-neurobiology-of-chronic-pain-to-enhance-patient-care/1271.

[xi] http://www.rupikaur.com.

[xii] *Huffington Post,* Emma Gray, "The Removal Of Rupi Kaur's Instagram Photos Shows How Terrified We Are Of Periods," 27 March

2015, http://www.huffingtonpost.com/2015/03/27/rupi-kaur-period-instagram_n_6954898.html.

[xiii] Endometriosis Foundation of America Nurse Conference 2013, Kimberly Smith-Niezgoda presentation, http://www.endofound.org/video/nurse-conference-2013-kimberly-smith-niezgoda-mac-lac-diplnccaom/412.

[xiv] Endometriosis Foundation of America Nurse Conference 2013, Kimberly Smith-Niezgoda presentation, http://www.endofound.org/video/nurse-conference-2013-kimberly-smith-niezgoda-mac-lac-diplnccaom/412

[xv] *WebMD UK Health News,* Nicky Broyd, "Endometriosis: Surgery lowers ovarian cancer risk," 10 April 2013, http://www.webmd.boots.com/ovarian-cancer/news/20130411/endometriosis-surgery-ovarian-cancer.

[xvi] *Journal for Healthcare Quality,* Johns Hopkins Medicine, "Hospitals Misleading Patients About Benefits Of Robotic Surgery, Study Suggests," 18 May 2011, http://www.hopkinsmedicine.org/news/media/releases/hospitals_misleading_patients_about_benefits_of_robotic_surgery_study_suggests.

[xvii] *Medical Daily,* Ed Cara, "144 Deaths Linked To Robotic Surgery In Past 14 Years: Are They Safer Or More Effective Than Conventional Surgeries?" 23 July 2015, http://www.medicaldaily.com/144-deaths-linked-robotic-surgery-past-14-years-are-they-safer-or-more-effective-344462.

[xviii] American Congress of Obstetricians and Gynecologists, James T. Breeden, MD, "Statement on Robotic Surgery by ACOG President," 14 March 2013, http://www.acog.org/About-ACOG/News-Room/News-Releases/2013/Statement-on-Robotic-Surgery.

[xix] *WebMD UK Health News,* Nicky Broyd, "Endometriosis: Surgery lowers ovarian cancer risk," 10 April 2013, http://www.webmd.boots.com/ovarian-cancer/news/20130411/endometriosis-surgery-ovarian-cancer.

[xx] American Cancer Society, "What are the key statistics about ovarian cancer?" http://www.cancer.org/cancer/ovariancancer/detailedguide/ovarian-cancer-key-statistics.

[xxi] Breast Cancer Research Foundation, "Breast Cancer Statistics and Resources," http://www.bcrfcure.org/breast-cancer-statistics-resources.

[xxii] The Yearbook of Obstetrics & Gynecology. Vol 6. Henry Reich. "Laparoscopic surgery for advanced endometriosis." Ed. PM Shoughn O'Brien. RCOG Press, London. Ch. 33. Pages 377-393. 1998.

Index

Note: Illustrations are indicated by *italics*.